What Others Are Saying About This Book

"...the most important lesson of the 21st century..."

"If there is one book you need to read to learn how toxins are making us sick and what to do about it, this is it. *Holler for Your Health* courageously says it like it is, and makes us take a serious look at the choices we make that contribute to our toxic environment. But more importantly, she guides us and empowers us with new choices to heal our bodies and our environment. She teaches us the most important lesson of the 21st century – that our health is intimately linked to the health of the planet."

-Mark Hyman, MD, New York Times best-selling author of UltraMetabolism and The UltraSimple Diet

"Every parent should read it."

"Teresa Holler has written with passion and commitment about one of the greatest challenges we face today: the environmental toxicity that threatens our present health, our families and our future. Teresa uses her medical background, her skill as a writer and her concern as a mother, to give us a thorough, practical book that guides its readers through all the steps needed to create safe environments. Every parent should read it."

-Leo Galland, MD, Author of the Fat Resistance Diet, Four Pillars of Healing, Power Healing, and Superimmunity for Kids

"...a powerful tool for parents..."

"Holler for Your Health is a powerful tool for parents to become aware, informed, and to take action. It should be considered essential reading for anyone interested in holistic healthcare, natural parenting, and non-toxic living."

-Nancy Massotto, Executive Director, Holistic Moms Network

"This is one of those books that every household should have."

"This is one of those books that every household should have. The content is captivating, extraordinary, and unbelievably believable. It is amazing what we don't know and even more incredible what is being kept from us, the consumers. I will be recommending this book to everyone I know. It doesn't matter what country in the world you live in, this book is relevant across the globe. Some of the content is shocking, frightening, inspiring, and is certainly a wake-up call to all of us to actually start becoming more aware of everyday things that we have just taken for granted as being "safe." This is not a book of conspiracy theories; it is a book of factual realities with clear and helpful tools to ensure the health and well-being of our families."

-Ruth Blaikie, New Zealand

"...valuable..."

"This book is quite valuable both to those starting out on their less-toxic journeys and also to those who are already well down the path."

-Beth Granai, Holistic Moms Network

HOLLER

for Your

HEALTH

Be the Key to a Healthy Family

Teresa Holler

First Edition

Healthy Harbor Enterprises, LLC

3

Holler for Your Health
Be the Key to a Healthy Family
By Teresa Holler

Published by:
Healthy Harbor Enterprises, LLC
http://www.healthyharbor.com

ISBN 978-0-9815261-0-2 First Edition 2008

Library of Congress Cataloging-in-Publication Data
Holler, Teresa.
    Holler for your health : be the key to a healthy
family / Teresa Holler. -- 1st ed.
    p. cm.
    Includes bibliographical references and index.
    LCCN 2008922023
    ISBN-13: 978-0-9815261-0-2
    ISBN-10: 0-9815261-0-1

    1. Toxicology--Popular works. 2. Environmental
health--Popular works.   I. Title.

RA1213.H65 2008   615.9
                               QBI08-600125

Dedication

In honor and in memory of all those whose lives have been
shattered by toxic chemicals.

And...

To the loving parents, grandparents, and guardians who are
arming themselves with the information needed to protect the
health of their children in an era where the potential for lifelong
health rests foremost in their own able hands.

And...

To my Sweet Sarah and Compassionate Chris

Foreword

"...a powerful tool for parents to become aware, informed, and to take action...it should be considered essential reading..."

-Nancy Massotto

Today's parents are increasingly aware of the challenges they face raising healthy children in a toxic world. From plastics to pesticides, children's growth, development, and health are in jeopardy. But rather than being paralyzed by fear, parents need to arm themselves with information and join together to support one another on their quest for health and well-being for themselves and their families.

Holler for Your Health: Be the Key to a Healthy Family is a powerful tool for parents to become aware, informed, and to take action. *Holler for Your Health* is an eye-opening book, alerting parents to the often overlooked risks of fluoride, mercury fillings, personal care products, and our food and water supply, among others.

But the book goes further by empowering parents to make changes by offering practical solutions and easy steps that we can all undertake to achieve a healthier lifestyle and reduce the toxins in our lives. It should be considered essential reading for anyone interested in holistic healthcare, natural parenting, and non-toxic living.

Become informed, support one another, and create change in your families and in our world community. If you are in search of other parents to support you along your journey to improved health and well-being, we invite you to discover the Holistic Moms Network at **www.holisticmoms.org**.

-Nancy Massotto, Executive Director, Holistic Moms Network

Preface

"I simply cannot stand by and watch parents lovingly poison their own children."

-Teresa Holler

You may wonder why I have written this book. Like everything in life, the answer is never simple. Those of you who are mothers, and perhaps fathers, may relate to the first reason. It is hard to explain, but once I became a mother I developed an instant emotional bond with all children. Any pain, loneliness, loss, or despair endured by any child became so much more poignant to me.

Several years later, while taking an environmental health course for my doctoral degree, I realized that I had been exposing my daughter to numerous toxins that were known to cause disastrous health problems. I was shocked to learn that toxic chemicals are hidden in numerous seemingly innocent household products as well as food and water. It occurred to me that if I had no idea of the dangers that lurked in my closets, pantry, and refrigerator, perhaps other people are as clueless as I. Perhaps people all over the world are unwittingly poisoning their loved ones just as I had been. How could someone without medical training be expected to know what I, as a medical provider for over a decade and instructor of the next generation of healthcare providers, did not? Thus, my passion for sharing this message was born. I simply could not and cannot stand by and watch parents lovingly poison their own children.

More people die from toxic chemicals than from motor vehicle accidents, and most of these exposures take place in our own homes. As we have immersed ourselves in products laden with hidden chemicals, society has become plagued with a host of chronic illnesses. In the span of one industrial century the incidence of cancer has soared from 1 in 8000 to nearly 1 in 2. In fact, nearly half of all Americans now suffer from at least one chronic illness.

The problem is obvious: toxic chemicals are bad for health and health is getting bad. Unfortunately, toxic chemicals are frequently omitted from labels, and grocery shopping now just about requires the shopper to have a PhD in chemistry. So, what can we do to preserve the health of our loved ones? *Holler for Your Health: Be the Key to a Healthy Family* reveals how to minimize exposure to toxic chemicals and increase the odds of remaining healthy in this era of illness.

Holler for Your Health is the product of nearly a year devoted to researching and filtering through a mountain of information so that the millions of people who do not have the luxury of time and a medical background may benefit from the information within. This is shared with the sincere hope that you, your loved ones, and especially your children, will lead happy, healthy lives.

Holler for Your Health begins by recognizing the inadequacies of relying on others to protect ourselves and our children. It then provides the information needed to avoid chemicals known or suspected of causing health problems. For instance, the following will be revealed:

☐ The scientific evidence regarding vaccinations and autism;

☐ The problem with silver dental fillings;

☐ Which plastic products are safe and which are not;

☐ What is in your drinking water and how to choose an effective water purification system;

☐ How to select less toxic food, children's toys, personal care products, cleaning supplies, cookware, and more.

Strategies to avoid toxins are offered to accommodate all families regardless of income. The book culminates in a 10-Step Action Plan to immediately apply this knowledge and achieve a lifetime of better health.

Holler for Your Health empowers each of us to take control of our own health rather than focusing on the institutions that are failing to protect us. The solution, to stop treating and start preventing disease, truly is in reach. It lies within each of us.

Thank you for reading this book. You truly can make a difference. Yes, you!

Acknowledgements

How fortunate I am to have the love of Chris and Sarah, who inspire me to try to make the world a healthier place. I love you both exactly as you are.

To my sister Sue who, despite overwhelming adversity, has grown into an extraordinary woman, mother, and friend. Thanks for just being you. To my sister Kathy, thank you for troubleshooting and late nights at the computer. You are appreciated more than you know! To Mom and Dad and Pat and Chuck, thanks for your support. To Mike, Steve, Kevin, and Aaron: you're the best!

Jeannye Sir, thank you for being a true friend and believing so strongly in my mission.

Sue Cuneo, thank you for your calming words and editing expertise when I needed it most!

Grace McGee is extraordinarily kindhearted; she has spent countless tedious hours selflessly editing and I am ever so grateful.

Alisa Callahan, although we may have been unable to see the purpose of our connection in college, it has become crystal clear in our maturity: to inspire and encourage each other on our paths to improve the lives of others. I am so glad we were given a second chance at friendship.

Pat Foreman, I am grateful in so many ways. Thank you for your friendship and willingness to join me on my quest.

Cathryn Harbor, Rebecca Katz, Mary Bahr, Kathie Swift, Kate Robinson, Lisa Dullaghan, and Nell Newman are extraordinary women who crossed my path at just the right time. They have inspired me or guided me along the way without being aware of how much it has meant to me. Thank you all.

To all who shared their heart-wrenching stories with me: thank you. Although I could not include them all, they touched my heart. Bobbie: your mother is most certainly smiling down upon you and your beautiful family.

To the extraordinary teachers at Pearl River High School and professors at Siena College: what a wonderful foundation you have given me both scholastically and personally. Thank you all.

And to those I have forgotten to mention, let's chalk it up to brain toxins and know that I wish you well.

Contents

Foreword
Preface
Acknowledgements

Section 4: Triumph Over Toxins

Section 5: Appendices

We Are the Answer

"Stop expecting Prince Charming. We must rescue ourselves. We are the ones we've been waiting for."
–Bella Abzug

While researching this book, I often became depressed by the atrocities committed against the environment and human beings of all colors, creeds, socioeconomic status, and most devastating of all, ages. It is hard to imagine that human beings in positions of authority could turn a blind eye to the harm inflicted on the most precious of all resources: our children. The chapters in this section are short by intention. The endless examples of ignorance, greed, and abuse of power are omitted so as not to result in outrage or a sense of hopelessness, which is not the intent of this book. Rather, it is my hope that it sparks a revolution of positive change by individuals united in one purpose: to prevent ourselves and our beloved children from harm.

After reading this section, I am hopeful that you will see that we need to redirect our energies. Our current institutions are failing to protect our children, but let's not waste precious moments gazing in the rear-view mirror, lest we become paralyzed by anger and despair. Let's focus on the power within each of us to make striking changes. The solution is within reach; it lies within each of us.

Chapter 1

A Toxic Soup

"There is nothing on this earth equal to, no nation has any resource greater than, the potential of just one child."
–Richard Pelzer, Author of *A Child Called It*

We all live in a toxic soup. We are bombarded with chemicals whose toxicity and potential dangers are often unknown. Although we may all suffer the effects of toxins, it is our children who are at greatest risk.

Children are uniquely vulnerable to environmental toxins. Their rapid metabolism, and growth and development expose them to more toxins by requiring increased consumption of food, water, and air for their body weight than adults. Children also behave differently from adults. They put everything in their mouths. Products may be considered to have "safe" amounts of toxins because they were not intended to be placed in the mouth. Crawling and spending more time on the ground places children in closer proximity to the toxins that settle in the earth and household dust. Toxins are also more likely to make a child ill because the systems required to detoxify or excrete these poisons are still maturing. Moreover, acceptable exposure limits are typically based on risk assessment calculations in adults, not more vulnerable infants and children.[1]

We now know that children are contaminated before they even take their first breath of air.[2] This is especially concerning because the blood brain barrier is not fully formed until months after birth allowing these toxins access to the brain where they may cause irreversible brain damage.

Brain Protector: The blood brain barrier shields the delicate brain from potentially harmful substances that may be circulating in the bloodstream.

Of the 287 industrial chemicals and pollutants found in umbilical cord blood from newborns tested in a 2004 study, 180 are known to cause cancer, 217 are toxic to the brain and nervous system, and 208 cause birth defects or developmental abnormalities.[2]

How did we manage to contaminate our children with all of these toxic chemicals before they have even taken a breath of air let alone smoked a cigarette? When we look at the information on toxic releases into our air and water, the answer is obvious. In 2004, US industries released over 70 million pounds of known carcinogens, 96 million pounds of known developmental toxins, nearly 38 million pounds of reproductive toxins, more than 826 million pounds of suspected neurological toxicants toxins and nearly 1.5 billion pounds of suspected respiratory toxins into the air and water.[3]

Yet these releases are not our greatest toxic threat. For every pound of these toxins dumped by New Jersey and Massachusetts industries, about 42 pounds are used in products intended for our homes.[4] In other words, *we* bring these toxins into our homes; our greatest toxic threat comes from our own purchasing decisions. This means we have the power to change the state of our health by simply choosing to purchase safer products.

Unfortunately this is no easy task. Chemicals known or suspected of causing health problems are frequently not labeled so consumers have no idea how toxic their homes have become or how to choose safer products. This book is intended to change that by providing practical tools and tips for making healthier choices. But first we need to understand that others aren't positioned to help. We must step up to protect ourselves.

Chapter 2

The Doctor is Out

"Each patient carries his own doctor inside him. They come to us not knowing that truth. We are at our best when we give the doctor who resides within each patient a chance to work."

-Albert Schweitzer, M.D.

Hippocrates is known to physicians as the "father of medicine." In his treatise, *On Airs, Waters, and Places*, he described how environmental factors, such as water quality, impact health status. Yet the message he began centuries ago is still largely ignored by those practicing conventional Western medicine. I should know; I am one of them.

While practicing medicine, I felt that something was missing. I entered the field of medicine to help people, yet I rarely felt fulfilled. It took me nearly a decade to realize what was wrong. I was unaware of a vast fund of knowledge that had been overlooked during my medical training.

Conventional medicine is brilliantly effective at treating trauma or acute illnesses. But when it comes to chronic diseases, this approach has failed. We have ignored centuries of knowledge as well as the successes of other cultures. I was not trained about preventing diseases nor was I successful in curing the chronic illnesses that plagued the majority of my patients. Neither was I, like the gross majority of other medical providers, familiar with the myriad of chemicals that people like Lydia are exposed to nor how these chemicals affect health.

Lydia is a chemist who works with noxious chemicals within pretreated wastewater before it is deposited into the local river. One day she began to notice symptoms that were unusual for her. Aware of a definite change in her body and knowing she was exposed to toxic substances, she feared that something could be wrong. Lydia sought help from a dozen medical providers before anyone heeded her cry. Finally, an insightful doctor took her environmental exposures seriously. Despite the fact that her symptoms may not have otherwise warranted it, the doctor ordered

15

a colonoscopy and identified several dozen precancerous abnormalities that should never have been found in such a young woman. Lydia was lucky she had been so persistent.

Unfortunately, Lydia is not alone. I used to cringe whenever a patient inquired about toxic exposures. I had no idea that toxic exposures impacted human beings or where to go to find more information. It is disconcerting to healthcare providers to be confronted with problems of which they know nothing about. Unfortunately, most conventional doctors are out of the loop on the role toxic chemicals play in illness.

Not Hostile, Just Untrained

If we are going to protect ourselves and our loved ones, we need to work together—not just with our peers, but with our healthcare providers. Conventional medical providers are often depicted as hostile toward alternative remedies. While this is certainly true of some providers, I believe most are open to other approaches to healing, but simply have little knowledge of alternative medicine and are uncomfortable suggesting or discussing that which they don't know.

This is certainly understandable in a litigious environment that uses current guidelines and standards of care to judge whether malpractice has occurred. Alternative regimens are rarely included in medical guidelines.

It is also difficult for doctors to find the time to learn new approaches when they are trying to keep up with an overabundance of information regarding new medications, drug interactions, and drug recalls in addition to seeing more and more patients in less time.

The Art of Medicine

When I was training to become a physician assistant I remember being taught that, "Medicine is an art, not an exact science." This statement reflected the individualized approach that was necessary to treat each unique person. Medicine has certainly changed course since I heard those words. Individual patients are now reduced to specific illnesses. Doctors are trained to make signs and symptoms fit into a particular diagnosis. Once this diagnosis is named, the patient is placed on a standard regimen without taking into account their uniqueness.

Contributing factors are frequently overlooked as well. For instance, if a patient complains of chest pain, the doctor will ask questions to see if the symptoms "fit" the pattern of risk for a heart attack. If so, the cookbook approach to care is followed. Since questions about chemical or pollution exposure are not part of the cookbook of questions, the underlying problem may never be identified. Is there any wonder that 50 percent of heart attacks are not a result of the standard risk factors and doctors have no idea why they occur?

It is because of these limits of the conventional healthcare system that patients are now seeking alternative remedies in escalating numbers. This is troublesome to those who profit from the conventional medical system. Perhaps this is the underlying reason for the new concept of Evidence Based Medicine (EBM) that is now being incorporated into medical education. The premise of EBM is that a medical provider's clinical judgment is not reliable and therefore, decisions regarding medical treatment should be made solely on the basis of medical studies. This cookbook approach fails to take into account that no company is going to fund a study on the benefits of a natural product that cannot be patented to produce billion dollar profits. EBM has effectively prevented physicians from endorsing more natural cures and maintains the edge for pharmaceuticals, which are substantially more profitable. Thus, the current system only promulgates courses of treatment that are well funded.

It also fails to acknowledge that many clinical studies are flawed by bias because they are funded by institutions that stand to gain billions of dollars in sales based on a favorable outcome and the methodology of scientific studies can be easily altered to create desired outcomes. This makes it crucial to know who is funding a study before deciding on its validity. Yet it has become increasingly hard to identify the funding of a study. For example, a recent study designed to prove that a chemical used in plastics was safe was conducted by the Harvard Center for Risk Analysis (sounds pretty non-biased, right?). But this study was funded by the American Plastics Council (sounds like a vested interest now, doesn't it?).

I have witnessed first-hand how patients taking a once popular arthritis medication arrived in the emergency room with worsening heart failure. My "gut feeling" told me something was wrong long before this product, with all of its great evidence, was pulled from the shelves. We have seen numerous drugs removed from the market or have additional warnings added to their labeling in the past few years. This highlights the fact that the evidence used to encourage the use of these products may have been flawed or deficient. Yet we are telling medical providers, who are making treatment decisions, to ignore what is right in front of their eyes and rely, instead, on flawed industry-funded studies.

Unfortunately, there is a great incentive to place dangerous products on the market. Even when a drug is discovered to cause illness and death, the manufacturer profits for as long as their product remains available for sale. As we will see in future chapters, the policy of placing dangerous products on the market to reap financial windfalls for as long as possible is seen in other industries as well.

Puppeteering

Healthcare providers have no control over the content of their medical training. Most have no say in the guidelines that they are following. Many have no idea who the "peer" reviewers are that decide which studies are published in the journals that they read to further their medical knowledge. They are unaware of the hand that controls their profession.

The majority of medical providers are not involved in the politics of medicine, but are busy working on the front lines trying their best to care for their patients. These concerned physicians are burning out in increasingly worrisome numbers. By not understanding why their patients are so sick, they are unable to make them well. Doctors are certainly overworked and increasingly underpaid, but this is not why they are burning out. It is largely because of the futility of current medical practices.

Closing the Gap

As patients, we are clinging to a failing medical system while reaching out for something better. Our insurance companies force us to use conventional medicine rather than alternative, often less costly, less invasive, and less toxic approaches. We have relied on conventional medicine for so long that we aren't sure who to entrust with our health, and we have difficulty finding reliable information upon which to base such an important decision. In essence, we are stuck in the gap between a medical system that has had many successes, but is now largely failing us, and an alternative means of healing, which may offer greater good, but is obscure, and in many cases, untested.

And so for now many of us are forced to depend on pharmaceutical products, which we know may inflict harm as well as healing. For now, we listen to our doctors half-heartedly, while inwardly questioning their medical advice. For now, we pick and choose which information we share with our doctors, while wondering if they will mock us for choosing to take herbs and supplements. For now, our overworked, frazzled doctors try to hide their irritation with those of us who question their logic, seek answers they cannot provide, and sidestep the use of their arsenal of feared treatment options. For now we are lost and unsure who to trust with our lives and the lives of our children.

Fortunately a new type of doctor has emerged, one that bridges the gap between current medical practice and alternative strategies by getting to the root of disease rather than treating or masking symptoms. This next generation of doctors includes Harvard trained physicians and a host of other traditionally trained practitioners who call themselves Functional Medicine providers. Their mission is to "improve patient outcomes through prevention, early assessment, and comprehensive management of complex, chronic disease.[1] To find a functional medical provider in your area, simply go to **www.functionalmedicine.org** and click on "Find an FM practitioner."

I am hopeful that the future of medicine will embrace a holistic and individualized approach to patient care and seek out ways to prevent rather than treat illnesses.

Chapter 3

*T*he Price of Proof

"There are three kinds of lies: lies, damn lies, and statistics."
-Benjamin Disraeli, former Prime Minister of Britain

Many people, including myself, have assumed that all products sold in American stores are safe. We shop with only our wants or needs in mind. Until I began researching this book, I never thought twice about buying make-up, lotion, baby shampoo, baby bottles, or teething rings. I even painted my daughter's room and allowed her to sleep in it the next night despite a lingering scent of paint. I never bothered to read the labels at the food store except to make sure there weren't too many calories or fat grams. And even if I had read each of the ingredients, how on earth would I have known what any of those ingredients were, or that they could be harmful? Most of us can't even pronounce the ingredients, let alone know what effects they have on our health.

We walk down store aisles in blind faith that our government has restricted the ingredients to those that are safe and that corporations would never produce and market products with the potential to harm us. Ignorance is blissful, but may be deadly. What I have learned is shocking, frightening, and for many families, devastating.

Time and time again, history has seen "the system" fail to protect us. This is true both here in America and all over the world. Industrial corporations benefit from the sale of deadly chemicals for as long as they can get away with it. To them, profit is the motivator and time is money. To us, time is the difference between life and death.

The strategy used by some corporations to keep dangerous chemicals on the market is simple: Deny, Delay, Discredit.

☐ Deny: When cancer and other illnesses are increasingly reported, simply state that it is a result of better detection rather than increasing rates of disease.

☐ Delay: Blame the victim. For example, if mothers would keep their homes cleaner then their children wouldn't get lead poisoning. This focuses resources on campaigns to change behaviors rather than focusing on the real issue of environmental exposure. Another delay tactic is to develop expert panels or call for more research in lieu of protective legislation or corrective action.

☐ Discredit: Hire scientific "experts" to find flaws in the research, conduct biased research, or claim there were other factors involved that resulted in the undesirable outcome.

"Magnifying or manufacturing scientific uncertainty is another tactic used to delay or prevent public health and environmental protection... Policy decisions should be made with the best available evidence and must not wait until every piece of evidence is in and until every conceivable doubt is erased."
-David Michaels, American Journal of Public Health, 2005

If the truth finally surfaces—despite the above tactics—some corporations have another trick up their sleeves. They state that they can't possibly comply with regulatory efforts to control toxic exposures or they will go bankrupt.

When air emissions standards for vehicles were first proposed, the American automobile manufacturers cried out that there was no way they could comply; the regulations would force them into bankruptcy. While they spent countless time, money, and energy fighting and delaying the implementation of environmentally protective legislation, the Japanese company, Honda, simply produced an automobile that met the standards.[1]

It is time we quit granting corporations extensions and provisions and open the market to those who can achieve results. We must level the playing field so that emerging American companies have the opportunity to excel. It certainly can be done. America is a land of innovation. If there is a need to be met, it will be met, but not when legislation ensures the success of corporate giants with questionable ethics.

President Nixon stated in 1970 that it was time that "America pays its debt to the past by reclaiming the purity of its air, its waters, and our living environment. It is literally now or never."[2] And yet here we are, nearly 40 years later, still poisoned in the name of economic prosperity. How many children have died, suffered, or have had their potential permanently reduced because of corporate delays and other tactics? We will never know because a system linking environmental hazards and exposures to health outcomes was not established until the Environmental Public Health Tracking Network emerged in 2004.

The Environmental Movement began because the public understood the problem of environmental degradation and they perceived the federal government as the only force powerful enough to improve conditions. There are good guys and bad guys in every discipline. When the bad guys hold key positions within the organizations that are supposed to be good, painfully little is accomplished. This is what went wrong with entrusting the federal government with the care and protection of the environment and our health. Such political debacles are not unique to the US. When dense fog claimed thousands of lives in London in the 1950s, an influenza outbreak was blamed to conceal the dirty truth that coal burning was the real culprit.[3]

General Motors, Standard Oil, and Dupont formed Ethyl Corporation in 1923 with the intent to market lead as an additive in gasoline. A brilliant marketing campaign convinced Americans of the benefit of this additive to combat the knocking noise in their cars while scientific "experts" reassured Congress that there was no proof of human health consequences from the manner in which lead, a known toxin to the brain and nervous system, was used in gasoline. When public health specialists from Harvard and Yale voiced their opinions that lead was unsafe in 1924, the Ethyl Corporation hired "experts" to refute this evidence. Such tactics succeeded in keeping leaded gasoline at American pumps until 1995.[4]

The effects of lead on the developing brain and nervous system of children are devastating, and yet we allowed lead to accumulate in the bloodstream of children at toxic levels for decades. Between 1976 and 1980, 88 percent of US children one to five years old had elevated levels of lead in their blood. One year after lead was completely phased out of gasoline, the percentage was reduced to less than 2 percent.[5] What will we say 70 years from now when we look back at the effect thousands of chemicals potentially more devastating than lead have had on generations of children?

In response to the accumulating body of evidence of the human health hazards of common chemicals, expert panels have been formed, research efforts expanded, and protective legislation hotly debated. And as all this deliberation, researching, and discussion has occurred, our health continues to be harmed. How many more young lives must be lost or limited? Must we continue to stand by and ponder whether the studies are conclusive enough or shall we wait until this sinister experiment has run its course through additional generations of unfortunate children? The price of absolute certainty is far too great. We are hiding behind the desire for definitive research. Would you take the support beam out of a house to see if it would collapse when common sense would suffice? We don't need more research, we need action.

Chemicals must be treated in the same manner as pharmaceuticals. They must be proven safe before they are unleashed upon the environment. Clearly, the chemicals that we breathe and absorb through our skin have the same potential for adverse reactions as those we intentionally ingest. Do we not administer medications like nitroglycerine in patches that are absorbed through the skin? Do asthmatics not inhale their medications?

I have read several well referenced books that describe in great detail all that I have touched on here. After reading them, I thought excitedly, "Yes! Now there will be a change. Now we will see the adoption of protective legislation." In each case I would then flip to the front cover and discover that the book was published many years ago. Protective legislation and sweeping cultural changes have not, in fact, occurred. Why has so little been done? Perhaps it is because we have relied on those in positions of authority rather than utilizing our greatest resource: ourselves.

Chapter 4

*F*riend or Foe

"...government is never more dangerous than when our desire to have it help us blinds us to its power to harm us."

-Ronald Reagan

As the public has grown weary of the toll that chronic illnesses and devastating diseases such as cancer have taken on themselves and their families, they have turned to charitable organizations and federal agencies in hope of finding a cure.

Charitable organizations claim they have increased their efforts at prevention and finding cures because that is what we, the public, are demanding they do. But their idea of prevention may be inadequate. Improving access to and quality of screening tests does not prevent illness; it merely identifies it in a more timely fashion allowing hope for a better outcome. While this is certainly beneficial for victims, they have already become victims. We don't want any more victims. We want healthy children, healthy parents to raise them, and healthy grandparents to love them.

Campaigns to improve lifestyle habits are an essential part of prevention, but such crusades portray the victim as responsible for their ill health and ignore other factors. If we truly want to improve health and prevent illness, there is another component of prevention that we are not addressing. Reducing or eliminating exposure to chemicals and pollutants in our air, food, water, consumer products, and workplaces is of paramount importance in preventing illness. Ignoring or belittling this fact is killing us. Unfortunately, both the National Cancer Institute (NCI) and the American Cancer Society (ACS) focus their initiatives on improved s, genetic research, and treatment while ignoring the of prevention unless it is a poor lifestyle choice. For an hind this misguided strategy read *Cancer-Gate: Losing Cancer War*, by Samuel Epstein.

When board members and large corporate donors of the organizations designed to protect us benefit from the proliferation of illness or the quelling of environmental concerns, they probably do not have our best interests at heart.

Cancer Charity Ratings: In 1992, *The Chronicle of Philanthropy* reported that the ACS was "more interested in accumulating wealth than in saving lives."[1] The ACS was rated with an abysmal one star for efficiency by Charity navigator.[2] Alternative cancer charities such as CureSearch National Childhood Cancer Foundation and the National Cancer Coalition both received four stars as an overall rating compared with two stars for ACS.[2]

Other organizations are failing us as well. The job of the Environmental Protection Agency (EPA), in theory, is to protect us from environmental hazards such as air pollution and water contamination. But the EPA does not conduct its own studies; it simply reviews the reports that manufacturers provide. The companies perform their own toxicity studies with little independent review.[3]

Instead of preventing exposure to known hazards, the EPA has developed a perplexing practice of determining "safe" levels of exposure to dangerous chemicals. How do they know what is safe? History, as in the case of lead, has shown that they do not. It is scientific guesswork at best, and a massive unethical experiment at worst. These scientifically determined "safe" levels provide a false sense of security. After decades of exposure, these "safe" levels are often proven to have been detrimental to human health. Acceptable levels are then unceremoniously reduced with no mention of the children and individuals whose exposures have already resulted in heart wrenching health effects.

Moreover, safety levels never take into account that in real-life, we are exposed to more than one chemical at a time. What effects do these chemicals have when mixed inside our bodies? We know that drug interactions can be deadly; so can chemical interactions.

Something has become crystal clear in the 50-year wake of the Industrial Revolution: there are no safe levels for chemical toxins. We just can't see the full extent of damage that lower levels of exposure cause. Barring a crystal ball, there is no way to introduce any new compound into an ecosystem or a human body and pretend that we know what the long-term effects will be. It simply becomes a clinical trial whose results may not unfold for decades or generations.

Another organization that is perceived to protect the public is the US Food and Drug Administration (FDA), which is responsible for overseeing the safety of foods, pharmaceuticals, and cosmetics. While there is no doubt they have done an excellent job of labeling the nutritional content of food, they have failed to disclose the ingredients or chemicals introduced to the food that are known or suspected to cause cancer, birth defects, or other illnesses. So while many of us painstakingly review labels to ensure a low sodium, low cholesterol product to prevent heart disease later in life, we have no idea whether they contain dangerous pesticides, plastic residues, or other hidden toxins, which may lead to far more devastating medical outcomes.

Moreover, the rash of pharmaceutical drugs removed from circulation because of safety issues or found to cause more harm than good is certainly an indicator of the danger that lies in assuming the US FDA has a clear vision of what is safe and what is not.[4] A few examples include the following:

☐ In 2003, the year before Vioxx was removed from the market, about 20 million Americans had taken this popular anti-inflammatory drug, which caused about 100,000 Americans to have heart attacks and 50,000 to die.[5]

☐ Baychol, the statin cholesterol lowering drug that is similar to Zocor, Pravachol, Lipitor, Crestor, Mevacor, Lescol, etc, was taken off the market after causing about 100 deaths due to a rare, but serious, side effect (rhabdomyolysis) causing muscle wasting and shut-down of vital organs. Half of the reported cases of this potentially deadly side-effect were reported with Baychol while the other half were reported by other statins, which remain frequently prescribed.[6]

☐ The once frequently prescribed allergy medications, Seldane and Hismanal, were removed from the market because their ability to incite abnormal heart rhythms resulted in several deaths. The deaths caused by these drugs were easily traced to their cause because the medications were often used by young, otherwise healthy, individuals. Many other drug-related fatalities go undetected because the patients are older, sicker, and the deaths are attributed to other factors.

☐   Of the millions of American women who took hormone replacement therapy, many chose to do so because they were told that it reduced their chance of having a heart attack. When this claim was finally tested in 2005, the results were alarmingly different than the advice touted by doctors for decades: women on hormone therapy had a 29 percent higher incidence of heart attacks and a 41 percent higher incidence of strokes. They also had a 26 percent higher incidence of breast cancer.[7]

"Federal processes (are) easily exploited by commercial interests to cloud the consensus about a toxicant's dangers."

–Dr. Herbert Needleman

It is difficult to know who to trust in this complicated web of deceit. Some industrial organizations have even started their own "charities" to control the course of research funds and manipulate the truth. There is no independent source to evaluate and regulate chemicals. Conflicts of interest abound. Are these conflicts to blame for losing the war on cancer and other chronic diseases? We may never know for sure. But one thing is certain, a lot of money has been spent and painfully little has been accomplished. There must be a better way.

Where shall we place our faith and hope for the right to a healthy life? Perhaps our money would be better spent by supporting grassroots organizations that are engaged in preventing environmental contamination rather than in organizations that fund the development of enormously profitable diagnostic and treatment products. After all, isn't it better not to get sick at all?

Chapter 5

Banding Together

"Alone we can do so little; together we can do so much."

-Helen Keller

Legislation hasn't protected us from harm; corporations don't always have our best interests at heart; some charities may have conflicting motives; and doctors aren't trained to recognize the impact of toxic chemicals or pollution on health. This certainly paints a bleak picture for those of us who are outraged that our children are poisoned even before birth. So what can we do about it?

Rather than focusing on what we can't do or the power that we lack, let us concentrate on what we can achieve and what power we possess. If we wish to succeed we need to work together. The strategy to divide and conquer is alive and well today. Having political parties forces us to choose sides and focus on the negative attributes of the other party, which prevents us from working together for the greater good. Let's respect each other's choice of political party, choose candidates who support our ideals regardless of their political affiliation, and focus our attention on what unites us rather than what tears us apart.

Perhaps when we realize that we are all on the same side—the side that protects young children and families, and that perhaps there is a darker force dividing us, we can begin to work together. We all want the same things; we all put our pants on one leg at a time (to borrow a saying from a Southern friend). We all make mistakes and are at different places on the learning curve, yet we all have the capacity to wake up each day and strive to do better. We must take care not to let the agendas of special interest groups fracture the inherent bond of human compassion and kindness.

Friend or Foe

We each have unique talents, gifts, and abilities. We can win the war against our real adversary, those who inflict harm for their personal gain. There is strength in numbers and there is strength in each of us. Let's learn about the toxic chemicals in our homes and then let's do something about it!

*T*he State of Our Health

"I am sick and tired of being sick and tired."
-Fannie Lou Hamer

Something has changed drastically regarding our health and well-being. Several generations ago, people endured the possibility of untimely deaths due to tragic accidents, acute infectious diseases, or childbirth. While these tragedies certainly took their toll on surviving loved ones, those who avoided such calamities seemed to live lives free of the burden of chronic pain or illness. In recent times we have seen a marked increase in diseases and syndromes that inflict prolonged pain and suffering, such as heart disease, cancer, diabetes, arthritis, and other degenerative diseases.

Chronic diseases are emerging as the most frequent cause of illness, disability, and death in America and other industrialized countries. Chronic illnesses are overwhelming our healthcare system and causing more and more Americans to forego increasingly costly health insurance. Annual medical expenditures are predicted to reach over one trillion dollars by 2020. Heart disease, stroke, cancer, and diabetes are examples of this new epidemic of prolonged human suffering, which has limited the lives of 125 million Americans and is responsible for 7 of every 10 deaths each year.[1] Nearly one half of all Americans suffer from at least one chronic illness.

The problem is not limited to adults. Chronic diseases are now replacing the infectious diseases as the leading causes of illness and death of children in developed countries. These illnesses are expanding in developing countries as well. Children are suffering from learning disorders, behavioral problems, mood disorders, asthma, allergies, and autoimmune disorders, such as multiple sclerosis (MS)—all in escalating numbers.

Children are now contracting chronic diseases that were once considered disorders only of adulthood. Doctors have renamed adult

30

onset diabetes as Type 2 diabetes because it is no longer an illness of adulthood. The most explosive growth of diabetes is occurring in the 15–19-year-old age bracket. The US Centers for Disease Control and Prevention (US CDC) believes that one in three US children who were born in 2000 will develop diabetes.[2] Diabetes is a leading cause of heart disease, stroke, kidney failure requiring dialysis, blindness, and lower extremity amputations. Now that diabetes is developing in younger patients, we can expect to see a dramatic rise in these and other illnesses at earlier ages than we've ever seen before. Today's children will be sicker and die younger than their parents.

Older Americans are not fairing well either; 80 percent are suffering from at least one chronic illness.[3] People turning 50 today are less healthy than those who have reached this age previously and doctors have little to offer the endless stream of patients suffering from chronic illnesses.

Through conversations with many of my patients I have come to realize that, with the exception of parents with young children, older people are not overly concerned about dying; they are worried about prolonged suffering and ill health. In general, people want to live a life free of pain, insomnia, depression, anxiety, doctor's appointments, surgeries, endless waiting for medical services, loss of independence, and diminished mental acuity. People are afraid of being chronically ill. Modern medicine is at a loss for what to do to prevent chronic illness and promote lifelong health, which has become a luxury of the past.

Yet poor health is not inevitable, with aging or otherwise. We can reverse this trend of prolonged suffering and pain. To do this, we must first understand the underlying reason for it. Poor lifestyle choices are rightfully receiving much attention as a contributing factor, but there is something else going on as well.

"Medicine is a social science. Don't we see that epidemics everywhere point to deficiencies of society?"
–Rudolf Virchow

History reveals numerous examples of the impact of social conditions on health and certainly should not be overlooked as we seek solutions to current medical enigmas. Squalor and overcrowded cities resulted in devastating epidemics of infectious diseases. The worst epidemics of the Black Plague were spread by the black rat, which thrived in squalor. Broad social problems may result in epidemics of disease while a social condition that affects a defined population may only afflict a cluster of people.

31

One example of a defined population becoming ill occurred when ships transporting people across the vast seas began to notice numerous deaths while en route. This perplexing problem was eventually attributed to scurvy, caused by a deficiency of vitamin C. Future deaths were avoided when lemons, limes, or sauerkraut were included in the ships' provisions.

A new epidemic has now emerged and the possibility of a new social problem must be considered and identified. If a social ill is unearthed and effectively addressed, these chronic diseases should be preventable. Much research has already linked many of these illnesses to a social problem: environmental toxins. Therefore, prevention of such illnesses should be easily accomplished through the implementation of appropriate public health measures. Unfortunately, sufficient measures are not uniformly in place. In the absence of such measures we will need to take matters into our own hands. We can educate ourselves and find ways to avoid the chemical toxins that contribute to illness.

This section reveals how toxins undermine our health and are often the root of a variety of illnesses. By avoiding toxins, we can all improve our odds of remaining healthy throughout our lifespan. It has been said that people only change when the pain of remaining the same exceeds the pain of changing. I believe the time has come.

Chapter 6

*D*efending Our Defenders

"Inflammation equals aging. Inflammation is the reason you get wrinkles; why you forget everything from where you left your car keys to your neighbor's first name; why you can be irritable and depressed and why you lose the healthy bloom of youth."

–Nicholas Perricone

Meet the Defenders

Each of us has an arsenal of defenses to protect us from illness. The skin and lining of our intestinal tract prevent foreign substances from gaining access to our bodies. The hair in our noses and respiratory tract, called cilia, catch foreign particles and carry them back toward the outside by waving them in that direction. Tears, saliva, skin oils, and stomach acid contain substances that kill bacteria.

These are all examples of barriers to prevent unwanted substances from damaging vulnerable cells and structures of the body. They are a part of the immune system that is designed to function properly immediately at birth. If foreign substances manage to surpass these first lines of defense, there is another protective system in place, the white blood cells. This vital component of the immune system is not fully developed until six months or so after birth.

A Balancing Act

The immune system must be perfectly balanced in order to function properly. A poorly functioning or weakened immune system can lead to increased susceptibility to infections such as colds, the flu, or recurrent ear infections.

While a weakened immune system is clearly undesirable, an overzealous system is no better. An overzealous immune system may begin attacking itself leading to autoimmune disorders or may cause chronic inflammation which leads to a variety of illnesses including Alzheimer's disease, heart disease, diabetes, and even obesity.

What is Inflammation?

Acute inflammation is a series of reactions triggered by injury or infection that culminates in heat, swelling, and pain. It is your body's way of trying to heal itself. While short-lived bouts of inflammation may lead to healing, *chronic inflammation* is like a smoldering fire that may damage any system or tissues within the body. Continuous exposure to a toxin or other irritant is a cause of chronic inflammation.

The reason many seemingly unrelated ailments can arise from one cause is complex, but is partially because of the interconnectedness of all the body's systems. There are nerves, hormones, peptides, and immune system cells all traveling around the body carrying messages and capable of spreading inflammation. This makes seemingly unrelated illnesses, such as asthma, allergies, inflammatory bowel disease, Alzheimer's disease, cancer, rheumatoid arthritis, and heart disease arise from one underlying cause: inflammation.

In addition to *spreading* inflammation, other bodily systems can also *initiate* inflammation independently of the immune system. For instance, when you smell a noxious odor, the nerve endings on your nose will release a chemical that leads to inflammation of the nasal passages causing you to sneeze or your nose to run. The inflammatory process may also extend to the lungs causing an asthma attack or may even trigger a migraine headache.[1]

When a baby suckles its mother's breast, tiny nerves in the breast relay the sensation to the pituitary gland where the hormone oxytocin signals for the milk to begin flowing. It is well known that a crying baby in another room can also cause a mother's milk to flow. How can this be? How does a baby that is away from the breast call oxytocin into action? Again, there is a vast network of communication within the body that includes all of our senses as well as our emotions. This just goes to show that the body is intricately connected and far more complicated than we can fully understand.

Just as many different bodily systems influence the immune system, the immune system influences more than just its own defense department. For instance, the immune system regulates thyroid hormone, which is vital in the development of the brain. When well orchestrated, such intricate connections keep the

34

body running smoothly. However, if even one bodily system is disrupted, a tangled mess of illness may result.

Immune Imbalance and Illness

Chronic inflammation afflicts more than 50 million Americans. It is a slow and silent killer. A study among the elderly revealed that frailty, increased blood clotting activity, muscle weakness, fatigue and disability were all linked to elevated markers of inflammation in the blood.[2] Inflammation is now surfacing as the underlying cause of a multitude of seemingly unrelated illnesses.

Inflammation has recently been accepted as a major factor in heart attacks, possibly more important than cholesterol levels, causing medical textbooks to be rewritten.

A young lady in her early forties with none of the traditional risk factors for heart disease came to see me for follow-up after having a massive heart attack. She did not smoke; she did not have high blood pressure, diabetes, or abnormal cholesterol and none of her family members had suffered from heart disease. When I began my career as a cardiology physician assistant, a Harvard trained cardiologist informed me that pre-menopausal women with no cardiac risk factors simply did not have heart attacks. But evidence to the contrary sat before me looking for answers.

My gut feeling was that something environmental must have contributed to her heart troubles. After asking her several questions that are not routine in the cardiology department, I learned that she had become a professional painter one year before her heart attack and had just finished painting when she had the actual event. Most paints contain volatile organic compounds (VOCs) that are emitted into the air where they are inhaled. These toxic compounds promote inflammation.

When I suggested that inhaling the toxic fumes from the paint may have induced an inflammatory response that led to her heart attack, she responded that she believed that to be true. The doctors at the hospital had dismissed this possibility, but she disagreed with them and was in the process of finding another line of work.

C reactive protein (CRP) is an inflammatory marker that is detected in the bloodstream. Elevated levels have been linked to increased rates of heart attacks and strokes, among other illnesses.

Inflammation has now been linked to the development of diabetes and some of its complications.[3] Inflammation of the intestines may lead to ulcerative colitis, diverticular disease, Crohn's disease, or other illness. These disorders are lumped together as "Inflammatory bowel disease" (IBD) and afflict nearly one million Americans each year. Recent evidence suggests that major depression is also associated with an abnormality of the immune system.[4]

It is now accepted that patients with advanced cancers often have underlying inflammation raging out of control. Indeed, chronic inflammatory conditions are major risk factors for developing cancer. In fact, anti-inflammatory medications such as aspirin have been found to dramatically reduce the rate of breast cancer in women.[5]

In addition to chronic inflammation, an overzealous immune system may begin to attack itself leading to a host of medical disorders called autoimmune disorders. According to the National Institutes of Health, 22 million Americans suffer from one of the 24 most common forms of autoimmune disease, and the numbers are rising.[6] In fact, the number one cause of disability among Americans over the age of 14 is arthritis or rheumatism.[7] Autoimmune disorders strike people down during the prime of their lives. Most cases are diagnosed between the ages of 20 and 40, although symptoms may have been evident long before a diagnosis is established. Although the site of destruction may vary, the root of the problem is the same: the immune system attacks cells belonging to "self". In MS, the insulation of nerves are destroyed while the joints are assaulted in rheumatoid arthritis.

Undermining Our Immunity

It seems that everywhere I turn nowadays I encounter another person complaining that they or their children are always sick. It seems that our immune systems have been compromised. In an article in *Environmental Health Perspectives*, Bob Weinhold reports that, "compared to just a century ago, there are hundreds of millions more people with weak or stressed immune systems."

Although there are many factors involved in the disruption of the immune system, the one that receives too little attention is the subject of this book: toxic chemicals. Continuous exposure to a toxin can cause chronic inflammation.

An example of this occurred in the families of leukemia victims in East Woburn, Massachusetts. Their continuous exposure to the toxins in their water supply overtaxed their immune system leaving them vulnerable to other infections or cancer.[8] In effect, their immune systems were so busy guarding the front door that there were no defenders available to guard against assailants who entered through the back. Blood tests confirmed this to be true: their immune systems were, indeed, chronically out of balance. This comes as no surprise given that trichloroethylene

(TCE), one of the chemicals responsible for this leukemia cluster, has been linked to the development of autoimmune disorders, which are known to result from immune system imbalance.[9]

Numerous other toxins have been associated with damaging effects on the immune system. Canadian wildlife biologist Peter Ross discovered that massive numbers of seals were dying off in the Baltic Sea because polychlorinated biphenyls (PCBs) had weakened their immune systems. The seals were simply no match for common viruses, which they once were capable of defeating.[10]

Immune dysfunction from PCBs has been seen in humans as well. For example, Residue from PCBs was dumped into an unlined pit in Anniston, Alabama, where it seeped into the groundwater. Those exposed to the contaminated water had an abnormality of their immune cells, which made them more susceptible to infection, autoimmune disorders, and cancer. Indeed, those exposed were said to have a high rate of "unexplained" cancer.[11]

In Denmark, researchers discovered that children with high levels of PCBs in their blood had a diminished ability to mount an immune response when vaccinations were administered. The effects of PCBs on the immune system were still apparent seven years later, indicating that PCBs may cause long-term damage to a child's immune system, leading to a host of medical problems later in life.[12]

Mercury has also been shown to produce an imbalance in the immune system leading to autoimmune disorders.[13]

> **"...mercury exposures quite below the average exposure can cause disruption of the immune system at all ages."**
> **–Boyd Haley**

Hormones also play a vital role in the proper functioning of the immune system. According to World Wildlife Fund scientist Theo Colborn, any substance that interferes with hormones can cause immune system imbalance.[14] Immune system dysfunction caused by hormone disruption may increase the risk of some cancers and autoimmune disorders. Unfortunately, we are bombarded with chemicals that disrupt this delicate hormone balance both before birth and throughout life. Hormone disruptors are discussed in detail in Chapter 7.

Getting to the Root of the Problem

When I was in college, I observed a curious link between autoimmune disorders and autism. It was a chance encounter with a woman who had severe lupus, an autoimmune disorder that can be crippling. Her lupus was so severe that she slept in traction. She needed assistance, and I was a poor college student in need of part-time work. I learned that her son suffered from autism, and that a friend of hers who suffered from severe rheumatoid arthritis also had a son with autism. As I was departing, she mentioned a book that was written by another victim of rheumatism raising an autistic child. My mind began to race as I began to see a connection between the two seemingly distinct ailments: autoimmune disorders and autism.

I ran to the library to search the literature. I could only find 11 citations in all languages. After reading all I could get my hands on, I developed a poster presentation for my class revealing the link between autoimmune disorders and autism. The A-plus I received was not what I was looking for. I wanted someone to see the connection; I wanted someone to do something about this amazing discovery; I wanted to prevent further illness!

Fortunately, scientists are now recognizing that inflammation may be the underlying cause of many seemingly unrelated illnesses. Although the root of this smoldering flame has many causes, the widespread exposure to toxins is one that is frequently overlooked. If we wish to eradicate chronic diseases, we must eliminate the toxins as well as the lifestyle factors that are undermining our immunity.

Chapter 7

Don't Shoot the Messenger

"Genes load the gun; the toxins pull the trigger."
-Unknown

It is commonly known that one's genetic code is responsible for one's medical and biological destiny. Genes are the blueprint for everything from eye color to temperament. But what is not as well known is that there is another factor within each of us that determines who we will become.

When building a house, the blueprint functions as its genetic code. It describes what the finished product is destined to be. However, the finished product may be quite different if the general contractor misinforms his subcontractors about how to complete the job. In the human body the endocrine system acts as the general contractor.

The chief players in the endocrine system are called hormones. Hormones are chemical messengers that travel in the bloodstream making sure that the genetic code is expressed properly. If the genetic code has an order, it is the hormones that see to it that it is carried out. In order to be born healthy and remain healthy, the blueprint must be correct and the orders must be correctly communicated to the individual cells, tissues, and organs of the body via the hormones.

Endocrine glands such as the ovaries, testes, thyroid, and adrenals release hormones, which carry their vital messages to their destinations. Some commonly known hormones are estrogen, progesterone, testosterone, melatonin, insulin, cortisol, and thyroid hormone.

Hormones are vital for normal development both before and after birth. The immune system, nervous system, including brain development, reproductive system, and numerous other processes rely on hormones arriving at the right place at the right time to facilitate their normal development and function.

The developing fetus is extremely sensitive to minuscule changes in hormone levels within the womb.[1] Because hormones are so incredibly powerful, these minute concentrations may be impossible to detect without specialized equipment, yet may dramatically affect the unborn child's development.

Health Effects of Hormone Disruption

There are chemical toxins in our midst that are capable of scrambling our hormones. These hormone disruptors masquerade as hormones as they travel throughout the body turning on, turning off, or changing the normal hormone signals. The end result is the disruption of numerous seemingly unrelated bodily functions.

Name Games: Hormone disruptors are also referred to as endocrine disruptors, xenoestrogens, xenobiotics or, because of their effects on numerous bodily systems, simply disruptors.

Chronic inflammation and immune system imbalance are just some of the detrimental effects of hormone disruption. Because hormones facilitate the interaction of all bodily systems, interfering with their messages may disrupt any bodily system.

According to a World Health Organization (WHO) report, hormone disruptors may adversely affect the nervous system and the reproductive system. By attacking the nervous system, hormone disruptors have detrimental effects on brain development, which may manifest as behavioral abnormalities, reduced intellectual capacity, or in physical abnormalities.[2]

Some of the effects on the reproductive system include impaired fertility, miscarriages, reproductive tract abnormalities, and early puberty. Hormone disruptors may also cause cancer of the breast, uterus, testicles, or thyroid.[3] A recent study suggests that high exposure to a hormone disruptor that leaches out of plastic products and aluminum cans may be associated with recurrent miscarriage.[4]

What is DES? DES is a manmade hormone, a synthetic estrogen, which was widely prescribed to pregnant women between the 1930s and 1970s to prevent miscarriages. It was later discovered to be both ineffective in preventing miscarriage as well as a trigger of vaginal cancer, birth defects, and immune system dysfunction in DES daughters.

Hormone disruptors may also be laying the foundation for what has become a dramatic social shift in modern culture: a growing transgender population. Perhaps hormone disruption plays a role in more and more people feeling they have been "born into the wrong body."

The science behind this theory is straightforward: the Y chromosome, which is carried in the sperm, directs the formation of the testes at just seven weeks of development. From that time on, it is the hormones released from the testes rather than the genetic makeup of the Y chromosome that directs the development of the rest of the characteristics that make a man masculine. If these hormones are interfered with at precisely the right time in development, a child born with a penis and testes may lack all of the other qualities associated with being a man.

Hormone disruption has already caused major aberrations of social behavior in animal populations. For example, birds exposed to hormone disruptors begin nesting with same sex partners. The females lose their maternal instincts leaving their offspring uncared for and vulnerable to predators and other threats.

Evidence now suggests that hormone disruptors may also be partly to blame for the current epidemic of obesity, diabetes, and heart disease. Hormone disruptors can lower testosterone levels; low levels of this hormone were linked to obesity, insulin resistance, and diabetes back in the 1990s. More recently, in 2007, plasticizers, which are known hormone disruptors, were specifically associated with an increased waistline insulin resistance, a precursor to diabetes.[5]

Several other studies back these findings. One study revealed a link between obesity and a hormone disruptor that leaches out of polycarbonate plastic. Another showed that mice that were given the estrogen mimic, DES, before or just after birth accumulated more body fat after they had reached puberty. Some also had a more difficult time processing sugar. Another study linked exposure to a chemical used in polyvinyl chloride plastics while still in the womb to a predisposition to gaining weight later in life.[6]

In 2000, The World Health Organization estimated that there were 300 million obese adults worldwide. Obesity sets the stage for numerous chronic health problems and may result in the bankrupting of our health care system. The preponderance of recent evidence suggests that current diet and exercise recommendations may be insufficient in thwarting this obesity epidemic. In order to combat the explosive growth of obesity-related illnesses the disruption of hormones must cease.

Hormone Disruptors Outnumber Hormones in Humans

As you can see, hormone disruptors are capable of inflicting a wide variety of ailments upon us. While it may be difficult to definitively link these agents to individual health complaints, there is no question that these hormone disruptors have invaded our bodies. Recent data shows that we have more hormone disruptors in our bodies than we have natural hormones.[7]

At the same time, the number of people suffering from health conditions linked to hormone disruptors has skyrocketed as the products containing hormone disruptors have gained widespread use. The products range from food and beverage containers, children's chew toys, personal products, and cleaning products. See Chapters 16 and 17 for details.

From this observation, we can surmise that if we avoid the substances that scramble our hormones, we may improve our health, our waistline, and effectively unburden our overwhelmed healthcare system. On a positive note, scientists have already identified several problem chemicals that have been linked to hormone disruption. Reducing your exposure to these chemicals by choosing healthier alternatives may improve your chances for good health.

Problem Products

Hormone disruptors come in a surprising array of everyday products. Everything from plastic chew toys, baby bottles, mattress covers, lotions, perfumes, detergents, shower curtains, ink, spermicides, sunscreens, IV tubing and other hospital supplies are potential hormone disruptors. It is not always easy to know if the products we commonly use are toxic to our hormones. But because of the serious health implications of hormone disruptors, it is imperative that we put forth the time and effort to limit the use of products containing these toxins.

Some of the hormone disruptors contained in the household products listed above include: commonly used plasticizers called phthalates (pronounced with a silent "ph"); a chemical that leaches out of polycarbonate plastic called bisphenol A (BPA); antimicrobial preservatives found in personal care products called parabens; and bromine-containing flame retardants. Additionally, pesticides and herbicides, heavy metals such as mercury, and other industrial chemicals such as PCBs and dioxins, are known to disrupt hormones.

Because hormone disruptors are pervasive in our present environment, you may become discouraged as you learn of all the toxic products you have used or exposed your family to. To prevent a feeling of hopelessness as you read on, take comfort in the fact that our body is designed to detoxify. In Section 4, you will learn how to support your body's natural filtration system in order to eliminate toxins. The next section will provide suggestions for healthier products. Small changes to your daily routine coupled with proper nourishment to strengthen your natural detoxification abilities, can make great strides in your lifelong health. So read on with hope rather than despair. You and your family can remain healthy in this toxic world, but you must first learn which seemingly harmless products are undermining your health.

Chapter 8

Neurological Nuisances

The nervous system, which encompasses the brain and spinal cord, governs our senses, mobility, speech, intellect, memory, mood, and decision-making. Our athleticism, musical skills, insightfulness, thought patterns, emotions, behavior, and personality all stem from a myriad of chemical processes within the nervous system.

When chemicals meddle with the nervous system, they can inflict a host of medical problems upon an individual while profoundly changing the social fabric of an entire species.

Degenerative Disorders

Degenerative nervous system diseases occur when nerve cells of the brain or spinal cord are damaged or destroyed. In addition to their involvement in movement, sensation, memory, and decision-making, nerve cells are also involved in communicating with and coordinating other bodily functions such as the cardiovascular system.

Alzheimer's disease, Parkinson's disease, Multiple Sclerosis, and other degenerative disorders may result from the destruction of nerve cells, which may have occurred long before symptoms develop. For instance, exposure to a toxin in childhood may destroy a number of nerve cells in the brain. However, the sheer number of remaining nerve cells may mask symptoms. As the child ages and more nerve cells are lost, he or she is at increased risk of developing a degenerative nervous system disease such as Parkinson's disease.[1]

Because neurons are not readily regenerated, reversing degenerative neurological diseases is unlikely once a significant number of cells have been destroyed. Prevention, through the reduction of toxic exposures, is of paramount importance.

Alzheimer's Disease

Alzheimer's disease is an all too common disorder that leads to dementia and death. It has been discovered that mercury exposure produces the same biochemical abnormalities found in Alzheimer's disease. A 1998 study found that patients with early

44

onset Alzheimer's disease had blood mercury levels that were almost 300 times higher than those who did not.[2]

What is Dementia? Dementia is a progressive decline in mental functions such as memory, attention, language, and problem solving. Alzheimer's disease is the most common cause of dementia. Reversible causes of dementia such as hypothyroidism, vitamin deficiencies, depression, and a condition called normal pressure hydrocephalus should be considered when someone develops mental decline. Normal pressure hydrocephalus has three classic symptoms: abnormal walking pattern, urinary incontinence, and dementia.

An inherited feature that leaves certain people vulnerable to mercury exposure is also involved in the development of this debilitating disease. There are two different versions of a protein that transports cholesterol out of the brain. One version is capable of also binding to and removing mercury while the other is not. The inheritance of the APO-E2 gene, which makes the protein that facilitates the removal of mercury from the brain, appears to be protective of Alzheimer's disease. On the other hand, the genetic inheritance of the APO-E4 gene, which makes the protein that is unable to carry mercury out of the brain, is associated with an increased risk of early onset Alzheimer's disease.

Parkinson's Disease

> **"The evidence that some environmental toxin or toxins play a role in causing Parkinson's is nearly unassailable."**
> **-Dr. Carolyn Tanner of the Parkinson's Institute**

Ten years ago my parents chose a great place to retire. They selected a walkable, historic downtown surrounded by beautiful beaches in a moderate climate. They developed a close friendship with another couple, Joe and Marilyn, who had retired there as well. Not long after they arrived, my father began getting sick with a variety of complaints that no doctor has been able to decipher. He complained of "pins and needles" and weakness in his legs as well as dizziness and other strange symptoms.

Several years later Marilyn was diagnosed with Parkinson's disease. I began wondering whether my dad and his friend were just following a natural course of aging or whether there was something in their new environment that led to their rapid deterioration upon relocating.

What is Parkinson's? Parkinson's disease, which afflicts up to 1 million Americans, is a progressively worsening neurological disorder characterized by impaired balance, tremors, difficulty with movement, and stiffness. The biochemical abnormality that results in these symptoms is the failure of nerve cells in the brain to produce dopamine sufficiently.

When I bumped into Marilyn at a wedding several months ago, she was no longer the same person. Her Parkinson's disease, or its drugs, had taken its toll. Her complexion was pasty, her personality flat, and her body was writhing rhythmically beyond her control. She looked miserable. She looked old. Two years ago she was neither of these things; she was a beautiful, feisty lady with an extraordinary sense of humor. What had happened to Marilyn?

I stumbled across a piece of information that made me suspicious of an unseen factor, which may have led Marilyn, and perhaps my father, to become ill. The beautiful town where they had chosen to retire lies in close proximity to a paper mill. Clusters of Parkinson's disease have been discovered among paper mill workers.[3] Paper mills, along with chemical companies, are the industries that release the largest quantities of nervous system toxins into the air and water.[4] Parkinson's Disease is a nervous system disorder.

The dizziness, weakness, and abnormal sensations experienced by my father are nervous system symptoms. Is it possible that exposure to these toxic releases may have contributed to Marilyn's demise and my father's misery? How could I ever prove this suspicion? Indeed, many top scientists have failed at similar tasks of establishing the cause and effect of environmental illnesses.

One thing I am certain of is that they both inhaled those toxins. You don't need scientists to prove that. Anyone living in the vicinity of a paper mill will agree that when you are downwind from the facility there is a distinctive odor. It is particularly noticeable on rainy days when you can actually "taste" it. But did this foul air cause their problems?

Unfortunately, we may never know. Marilyn, like the majority of people diagnosed with Parkinson's disease, is said to have "idiopathic" disease, a fancy medical term meaning the cause is unknown. Perhaps the cause is unknown because we are not asking the right questions.

Medical providers are not trained to ask questions about environmental exposures and if we do not ask the correct questions we certainly will not find the answers. In my father's case, he did have an astute physician inquire about toxic exposures. He was tested for arsenic and several other toxins. But with over 100,000 chemicals in the environment and unknown effects caused by their interaction with each other within our bodies it is impossible to test effectively. He remains undiagnosed and untreated.

Deadly Combinations: Scientists at Tulane University discovered that a mixture of pesticides is hundreds of times more toxic than an individual pesticide. This may explain why many chemicals, when tested individually, have not been linked to Parkinson's disease or other illnesses. Many more chemicals may cause illness if their exposure is in combination with other toxins that increase a person's vulnerability to that toxin. For example, University of Rochester scientists have studied an antifungal that is used in farming, called maneb, in combination with pesticides. Because maneb causes imbalances to the body's antioxidant defense system, exposure to it results in impaired detoxification and therefore, increased vulnerability to other toxins. Maneb remains on produce even after it is washed.[5]

Let's take a closer look at "idiopathic" Parkinson's disease. The first clear description of Parkinson's disease was recorded by James Parkinson in 1817, which correlates with the beginning of the Industrial Revolution. Since this time it has become a common observation. William Langston of California's Parkinson Institute believes that this coincidental timing "...raises the very interesting question... could it be a true manmade disease? A disease that was the result of something we introduced into our environment?"

The first incident supporting his theory that a chemical may be causing this new affliction occurred when young heroin addicts in Northern California injected a "designer drug" intended to mimic heroin. Unfortunately, the compound they ended up taking was MPTP, an industrial chemical. The unfortunate young addicts rapidly developed all of the classic symptoms of Parkinson's

47

disease, which is usually a slowly progressive disease seen in older people. Researchers discovered that the chemical caused the Parkinson-like symptoms by attacking the very same part of the brain as traditional Parkinson's disease.

Studies with twins then strengthened the theory that chemicals are involved in Parkinson's disease by suggesting that genetics play a minor role while environmental factors carry the bulk of the blame.[6] Additional evidence confirms that nervous system toxins cause the same biochemical abnormalities found in the disease.[7]

The chemicals that are most strongly suspected in Parkinson's disease include heavy metals such as manganese or iron, PCBs, solvents, certain pesticides and herbicides, and hormone disruptors. Prescription anti-psychotic medications are also known to cause a "Parkinson-like syndrome."

Persistent Problems: Although PCBs were banned in the US in 1977, they remain widely prevalent in the environment because of their persistence. They accumulate in the food chain and are a common contaminant in seafood. They are stored in fat tissue such as the human brain.

Chemicals suspected of causing Parkinson's disease include the following:

☐ Heavy metals: Manganese has caused parkinsonism in people who were exposed occupationally.[8] Iron has also been implicated in Parkinson's disease.

☐ PCBs: These alter dopamine levels, the brain chemical known to be involved in Parkinson's Disease.

☐ Solvents: These are also implicated in Alzheimer's disease and Lou Gehrig's (Amyotrophic Lateral Sclerosis) disease.[9]

☐ Pesticides/herbicides: A large study showed that people exposed to pesticides had 70 percent more Parkinson's disease than those who were not.[10] Studies have also confirmed an increase in Parkinson's disease in people who have been exposed to agricultural chemicals. People who drink water from shallow wells are more likely to be afflicted as well. This is believed to result from pesticide contamination from nearby agricultural sources.[11] At least one herbicide has been shown to destroy the same nerve cells that are ravaged by Parkinson's disease.[12]

☐   Hormone Disruptors: One of the effects that hormone disruptors have on the brain is to alter dopamine levels, which is the same biochemical problem seen in Parkinson's disease.

☐   Prescription anti-psychotic medications: These may cause a "Parkinson-like syndrome."

Parkinson's disease likely results from more than one factor. For instance, a genetic susceptibility may render a person particularly vulnerable to developing Parkinson's disease if they exceed a certain threshold of toxic exposure from one or many sources. Each person's lifetime exposure to a plethora of toxins along with their individual ability to detoxify and their individual susceptibility for certain diseases likely determines who gets sick and how their sickness manifests.

In Marilyn's case, the paper mill spewed out far greater quantities of nervous system toxins than any other polluter in her area. Nearly five million pounds of nervous system toxins, such as methanol, ammonia, and other chemicals are emitted from the typical paper mill. Methanol is known to cause nerve damage as well as headaches, vision disturbances, blindness, lack of muscle coordination, and even death.[13] Because methanol takes a long time to be eliminated, each exposure has additive effects on the body. The cumulative effect of these nervous system toxins along with other toxins that may have accumulated over her lifetime may have exceeded Marilyn's detoxification abilities, pushing her over the edge from wellness to sickness.

Perhaps the subtle nervous system complaints experienced by my father are another manifestation of the same chemicals emitted from the paper mill. Or perhaps both of their symptoms would have occurred regardless of their proximity to the paper mill.

How to Reduce the Formation of these Toxins: Limit the use of disposable paper products and purchase only unbleached paper products.

Multiple Sclerosis

Although most experts believe that MS is an autoimmune disorder, it is discussed here because it is also a degenerative neurological disorder. In MS, the insulation of nerve cells is gradually destroyed. This interferes with the conduction of nerve signals resulting in a wide variety of symptoms depending on which signals within the brain and spinal cord are impeded. Symptoms may come and go and include pain, visual problems, muscle weakness, abnormal sensation, depression, severe fatigue, incoordination, trouble balancing, difficulty thinking, and speech defects. Severe cases cause permanent disability.

MS is the most common debilitating disease that afflicts young adults in the prime of their life (20–40 years of age). As with other autoimmune disorders, MS is more common in women than in men.[14] MS is chronic, progressively worsens, and has no known cure. Therefore, prevention is of vital importance. In order to prevent MS, we need to discover what causes it. MS is not considered to be a genetic disease, although genetic factors predispose certain individuals to developing it.

Genetic Link to MS: People who inherit the HLA-DR2 antigen are genetically at higher risk of developing MS.

One clue that genetics are not solely responsible for MS is that when people migrate from an area with a low rate of MS to an area with a higher rate, their children assume the higher rate of risk associated with their new home. Clearly, something in the new environment contributes to this difference.[15] Several studies have shown that when children migrate before the age of 15 they acquire the new region's risk of MS, but if they do not relocate until after the age of 15 they retain the lower risk of their homeland. Such observations imply that environmental factors during childhood may cause damage that results in the development of MS later in life.

So what environmental factors are involved in MS? Those who suffer from MS have a wide variety of symptoms and level of disability making MS more a motley collection of symptoms rather than a disease state. Perhaps this disease of many manifestations is also a disease of many causes.

Some evidence, including a geographic preponderance of cases in climates with limited sunshine, suggests that lack of Vitamin D may be linked to MS. This link was recently confirmed by a large study by the Harvard School of Public Health. The further a person lives from the equator, the greater their risk of developing MS.

Evidence is also emerging that certain toxic exposures mimic the disorder and may contribute to the development of the disease. Because Vitamin D is required for the proper functioning

of the immune system, an inadequate supply may predispose
people to MS if they are exposed to toxic triggers.

Sources of Vitamin D: The body cannot manufacture Vitamin D
and dietary intake is minimal. Sufficient sunlight or
supplementation is essential for insuring an adequate supply of
Vitamin D.

Studies are beginning to suggest that one of those toxins is
mercury. According to Patrick Kingsley, of the nearly 4,000
patients with MS that he has treated, only five did not suffer from
mercury toxicity. In a recent Swedish study, the spinal fluid of MS
victims had six times the level of mercury of healthy individuals.[16]

Vitamin for MS? MS patients typically have far lower levels of
Vitamin B12 than healthy people.[17] A small study found that
supplementation with vitamin B12 improved several MS patients'
ability to see and hear.[18] This study requires further research, but
provides hope for a reversal of symptoms in a disease once thought
to be incurable.

Mood Disorders
Proper levels of brain chemicals are essential to our mental
health. Yet poor nutrition, stressful lifestyles, and toxic chemicals
have undermined the levels of these chemicals in an alarming
number of people.

Depression
Depression is a major health problem with nearly one of five
people having depressive symptoms at any given time. Depression
may manifest as disinterest (apathy), anger, hatred, self-mutilation,
eating disorders, or suicide. Teens may mask their depression by
withdrawing into their inner selves, becoming sexually
promiscuous or using mind-altering substances such as drugs or
alcohol.[19]
There are many factors underlying the development of
depression. Studies in twins show that there is a genetic
component in many mental disorders, but that markedly different
outcomes can result from the same genetic make-up. For instance,

in more than 50 percent of cases, identical twins who share the same genetic make-up do not share the development of the disease.[20] Once again, environmental factors are involved.

In the general population, twice as many women than men suffer from depression. However, in the Amish population in Pennsylvania, the rate of depression is equivalent in men and women and is much lower than the general population. Based on this information the Surgeon General concluded that "Something about the environment thus appears to interact with a woman's biology to cause a disproportionate incidence of depressive episodes among women." Since depression is known to be associated with abnormalities of immune system cells, it is possible that hormone disruptors, which are known to impair immune system function, may have a role in causing depression.

Below are examples of some chemicals that have been linked to depression:

☐ Pesticides: In the developing brain, serotonin systems are among the most sensitive to disruption by pesticides known as organophosphates.[21] Serotonin is the target of the most commonly used antidepressant drugs. Although banned in 1987, the once commonly used termite treatment, chlordane, has been associated with mood disorders and psychological problems.

☐ Rocket Fuel (Perchlorate): This interferes with the production of thyroid hormones. Lower levels of thyroid hormones can cause depression, anxiety, fatigue, and sexual disinterest.

☐ Mercury: When describing the symptoms and signs of occupational mercury poisoning, a 1771 author mentioned the "unusually sad mental state of these workers."[22] Long-term occupational exposure to mercury has been associated with depression, irritability, introversion, apprehension, loss of self-confidence, and other nonspecific symptoms.[23]

☐ Stress and dietary factors also contribute to depression.

Stress

The pituitary gland is often referred to as the "Master Gland." In reality, the pituitary is a puppet on strings and the strings are pulled by the hypothalamus. The hypothalamus is located within the brain, but is not protected by the blood-brain barrier, leaving it vulnerable to dangerous substances traveling in the bloodstream. The reason the hypothalamus is left exposed is that it requires continuous access to the messengers circulating in the bloodstream. It monitors the levels of these messengers in order to regulate bodily functions.

When toxins are present in the bloodstream, the hypothalamus identifies this as a stressor to the body, similar to other common stressors, such as pain, trauma, emotional upset, sleep deprivation, infection, and low blood sugar. The hypothalamus responds to these stressors by signaling the release of cortisol. In ancient times, cortisol was released in times of famine and other severe stressors in order to insure a constant supply of blood sugar (glucose) to survive.

Our environment has changed rapidly from a time of famine to a time of abundance; from a time of infrequent, life-threatening stressors to a time of continuous, trivial stressors. The hypothalamus has not had time to adapt to such dramatic changes. This means that the chronic exposure to low-levels of toxins, which is perceived by the hypothalamus as a stressor, results in the continuous production of cortisol.

The continuous, rather than intermittent effects of cortisol, have detrimental effects on virtually all bodily systems. Cortisol insures a constant supply of glucose, which leads to obesity and diabetes. This then leads to an increased production of masculine hormones, which may cause polycystic ovarian syndrome and male pattern hair growth in women.

Because the presence of cortisol signals that a threat is imminent, the body concentrates on survival at the expense of the "luxury functions," such as sex, digestion, and growth. This is why chronically stressed individuals lose their desire for sex. Stress causes decreased digestion in the stomach accompanied by increased transit through the colon. This means that there is less time for nutrients to be absorbed into the bloodstream, leading to nutrient deficiencies. The ensuing inflammation of the digestive tract leads to a "leaky gut," which allows more toxins to access the bloodstream and leads to sensitivities and allergies to common foods that were once well tolerated.

Aldosterone is another hormone released in stressful times. Aldosterone is responsible for increasing the volume of blood in circulation in order to supply sufficient oxygen for the fight or flight response. It accomplishes this by increasing the amount of sodium (salt) retained by the kidneys. When sodium is retained, so is water. Unfortunately, the chronic presence of stress, in the form of toxins or otherwise, leads to chronically elevated blood volume, which causes high blood pressure.

The hypothalamus also signals the fight or flight nervous system in times of stress. This causes an increased heart rate, anxiety, rage or stress-induced fighting, aversion to taste, increased startle response to noise, and irritability.

Cortisol also depresses the immune system leading to the development of numerous other diseases. Chronic exposure to toxic, or other, stressors forces the adrenal gland to continually supply cortisol. In time, the adrenal glands burn out, contributing to chronic fatigue syndrome, fibromyalgia, post-traumatic stress disorder, post-partum depression, and depression.

Avoiding toxic stressors may prevent some of the symptoms or diseases listed above. If avoidance of toxins or stressful situations is impossible, relaxation methods such as deep breathing exercises and yoga will help lower cortisol levels.

Can Detoxification Alleviate Depression? In the aftermath of the World Trade Center tragedy, many of the rescue workers succumbed to depression. The scope of the tragedy coupled with the carnage they were exposed to while searching for survivors and cleaning up the site certainly would be a likely cause of depression. But toxins may have also contributed to the undermining of their mental health. It has been established that the dust inhaled by rescue workers contained nervous system toxins. Rescue workers who participated in a detoxification program, which is discussed further in Chapter 22, had dramatic improvement in depressive symptoms.

Suicide and Homicide
The standard American diet is highly processed, loaded with chemicals, and deficient in vital nutrients. The horrifying way we eat may be contributing to the rash of heinous crimes, school shootings, and teen suicides we have been witnessing in recent times.

Suicide
A study conducted by the University of North Carolina at Chapel Hill suggests the possibility of a link between toxins in the air and an increased rate of suicide. The study demonstrated that during the time that operations of a nearby paper mill had changed, a sustained elevation of the suicide rate occurred. The operational change involved burning chlorinated compounds, which is known to release toxins such as dioxins and hydrogen

sulfide. A similar suicide cluster in a second North Carolina county was also linked to air pollutants released from several industries, including another paper mill.[24]

When chemical and wood waste (called "black liquor") is burned to generate electricity, hydrogen sulfide and other chemicals are released. In animal studies, hydrogen sulfide has been shown to be a nervous system toxin. Human exposure to occupational levels of hydrogen sulfide can result in nervousness, mania, dementia and violence.[24] A study of the causes of death among workers in certain mercury mines revealed an increased death rate due to suicide among the miners.[25]

The rate of suicide has skyrocketed since the 1950s, propelling it into position as a leading cause of death among US youth. It is time to consider the role of toxic chemicals in this epidemic.

Homicide

The homicide rate is higher among youth in the US than any other developed nation. It is the number one cause of death in African American males between 15 and 24 years of age and the second leading cause of death in all teens 15–19 years of age.[26]

Social defects are one of the risk factors for homicide. Such defects have been attributed to toxins in the environment. In essence, we need to clean up our act environmentally before we will have much success in cleaning up the behavior of violent criminals.

In animal studies, aspartame, which is commonly found in soft drinks and sweets, led to a roller-coaster ride for the brain chemical known as tryptophan. After a dramatic elevation, it quickly plummeted. Low tryptophan levels have also been linked to violent and aggressive behavior. When junk food and sugary drinks were replaced with fruit juice and fresh fruit or nuts, assault and battery among jailed criminals dropped 82 percent.[27]

Not So Sweet: Aspartame (Equal, NutraSweet), a common sweetener in "diet" foods and drinks, causes an increase in cancer risk even at doses much less than the current acceptable daily intake.[28]

Attention Deficit Disorder (ADD)

Millions of children have been diagnosed with attention deficit disorder or attention deficit hyperactivity disorder

(ADD/ADHD). The number of cases of ADD has escalated dramatically over the last decade resulting in a generation of children who have been prescribed stimulants such as Ritalin, despite lack of studies to determine their long-term safety in children.[29] Are there alternatives to these medications?

Many researchers believe there are. In the 1970s, Dr. Benjamin Feingold stated that he had improved symptoms in 30–50 percent of hyperactive children by simply changing their diet. In 1975, a committee of the US Department of Health, Education, and Welfare stated that Dr. Feingold's findings were sufficient to warrant further investigation about the impact of diet on hyperactivity. In 1982, the National Institutes of Health concluded that food additives and certain foods affect some children with behavioral problems. Although they recommended more research, they failed to sufficiently fund such efforts. Fortunately, other scientists in the US, Canada, Europe, and Australia conducted additional studies; 17 of 23 of these studies revealed significant worsening of behavior in children as a result of certain foods.[30]

While it is unknown what percentage of children with behavioral problems will benefit from dietary changes, it is certainly reasonable to try dietary modifications prior to initiating medications, which have no guarantee of long-term safety in children.

Amphetamines (Adderall, etc), along with their cousins the methylphenidates (Ritalin, Concerta, etc) are the primary treatment strategy for ADHD. These drugs exert a potent stimulating effect upon the central nervous system. Numerous children become plagued with a permanent side-effect known as Tourette's syndrome, which causes embarrassing tics. Affected children may display a variety of involuntary and socially devastating behaviors, such as lip smacking, tongue thrusting, moaning, hitting themselves, arm flapping, obscene gestures, and other repetitive actions. Although some fortunate children will recover spontaneously, there is no known cure. Treatment is with antipsychotic drugs like Haldol; the same drugs once used to sedate demented patients in lieu of tying them to the bed with restraints.

ADHD drugs also stimulate the cardiovascular system. They increase heart rate and blood pressure sufficiently to cause an increase in heart disease and death. The US FDA added a warning label in 2006 regarding the risk for cardiovascular complications with these medications.[31]

A study by the National Toxicology Panel linked Ritalin to liver tumors in rats. The US FDA claimed this was only a weak sign of cancer-causing potential with Ritalin and maintains its safety. However, waiting to see if the millions of children exposed to Ritalin will indeed develop liver cancer will take decades. The US FDA's Drug Safety and Risk Management Advisory Committee agree that prescribing these drugs to millions of Americans is inappropriate.[32]

Making dietary changes avoids the potential for serious risks and costs nothing, but is rarely presented to parents as a treatment option. [33]

Pumpkin Seeds and ADHD: Nutrient deficiencies have also been identified in children with ADHD, particularly magnesium. One study showed that a six-month regimen of magnesium supplementation resulted in a significant decrease in disruptive behavior.[34] The best food sources of magnesium are roasted pumpkin or squash seeds. These can be added to cereal, smoothies, shakes, yogurt, or eaten right out of the hand.

Chapter 9

Mind Games

"We are conducting a vast toxicological experiment in our society in which our children and our children's children are the experimental subjects."
-Pediatrician Herbert L. Needleman

Nervous system problems typically take years to manifest. This is why most of the degenerative disorders of the nervous system appear late in life. Unfortunately, with toxic exposures occurring very early in life, even before birth, children are now suffering from the effects of damaged nervous systems.

The number of children under the age of 18 in the US suffering from one or more learning, behavioral, or developmental disabilities is estimated at nearly 12 million.[1] Since 1971, the number of children taking Ritalin has approximately doubled every four to seven years. Further, the number of children in special education classes due to learning disabilities increased 191 percent from 1977–1994.[2] Such dramatic increases in disorders of the mind reflect a rising epidemic among children.

Experienced teachers will attest to the increased difficulty in dealing with today's students. Many cannot sit still, cannot concentrate, and are often disruptive or violent. Others have difficulty processing information and some are afflicted with more serious disorders, such as autism.

Children are now contaminated with toxins that damage the nervous system and brain development before birth, so it is not surprising to see these ailments in today's youth. Our children have lost the right to be born healthy.

The Developing Brain
Unborn children and young children are uniquely vulnerable to nervous system toxins because their brains are still developing. Most of the brain's cells are developed while in the womb. This requires extraordinary precision. All of the messengers must arrive in the correct time-frame and sequence in order for the

brain to develop properly. If any of these crucial steps are delayed or interrupted, permanent damage may occur. The placenta, which provides nutrition to the growing fetus, inadvertently facilitates the passage of toxins from the mother to her unborn child. Unfortunately the blood-brain barrier is not fully functional until several months after birth, leaving the unborn child's brain extraordinarily vulnerable to environmental pollutants passed on from the mother to the child.

Once a child is born, the brain continues its rapid maturation over the next several years. If the child is exposed to toxins at such crucial stages in development, irreversible damage may occur. Such defects may be immediately apparent or may not manifest until the child reaches maturity.

Studies reveal that a wide range of industrial chemicals that confer no harm to mature brains may cause toxicity to developing brains even at low doses. These chemical toxins may lead to brain disorders such as autism, attention deficit disorder, mental retardation, and cerebral palsy, which can all cause lifelong disability.

One in six children now suffers from a developmental disability and most of these involve the brain or nervous system.[3] Most of these disorders are said to have unknown causes, yet a diverse assortment of toxic chemicals in the environment is capable of causing these disabilities. Metals, solvents, and pesticides are among the greatest threats to the developing brain. Exposure to low levels of these chemicals during early fetal development can cause permanent brain injury. An additional 200 chemicals known to affect the mature brain are in use yet have not been studied to determine their effects on the more vulnerable developing brains of children.[4] It would certainly seem that the developing brain would be far more able to function normally in the absence of such chemicals.

The Subtle Effect

Developmental toxins may also exert subtle, so-called "subclinical" effects. Such a term implies the effect is not significant enough to cause an obvious problem. But just because it is not obvious does not mean it does not place a substantial burden upon the affected individual and society.

Learning disabilities result from scrambling of information as it travels from the senses to the brain. This results in individuals with normal or above-average intelligence having difficulty with retaining, processing, and expressing information. According to Jane Browning, Executive Director of The Learning

Disabilities Association of America, "As many as 10 percent of the school-aged population may have learning disabilities... even though these are smart and sometimes even gifted students, they often fail in school and must struggle with their learning disabilities throughout their entire lives."[5]

Below is an account of a smart, observant, and wonderful man with a learning disorder, as told by his wife:

> Chris has a learning disorder. He has never been formally diagnosed, but has certainly been greatly affected by it. When he was in college, I read his literature assignments aloud because he was unable to process the information by reading it himself and it would take an enormous amount of time for him to complete. Many words were beyond his comprehension and needed to be interpreted for him. When he read himself, words would become garbled and nothing made sense.

> When we were first married, I used to get frustrated with him because I would request three items from the store or ask him to run three errands. He would invariably return with only two items or complete only two of the tasks. He would then berate himself for being "such an idiot." We soon realized that his mind could only process two items at a time. We overcame this problem by using lists. He has to write down every chore or request so as not to forget.

> Because of my husband's difficulty processing information, he has had poor luck finding meaningful work. He lasted only one day as a waiter because he couldn't enter the customers' orders into the computer. The cash register defeated him at a retail position. He was unable to pursue his dream of being a gym teacher because he failed the national certifying exam three times. A firefighter exam got the best of him as well. He failed out of an EMT program despite answering every question correctly when I verbally quizzed him before the exam.

> Can you imagine the effect all of this failure has on a person? His self-esteem is in constant need of repair. We have opted for him to become a stay-at-home dad after some negative experiences with our daughter's daycare. The fact that the last job he

applied for offered only minimum wage was also a contributing factor in that decision. After taxes and daycare expenses we would have been spending money to send him to work. Besides he wasn't even offered the job. The company knew that high school students were better suited for these low wage jobs.

Although the cause of Chris's difficulties may never be known, there are some chemicals that are highly suspect. Let's take a look at some of the toxins that are imposing enduring limits on our children's abilities:

☐ Mercury: Mercury is particularly harmful to the developing brain. The Learning Disabilities Association of America (LDA), the National Education Association (NEA), and the Arc of the United States claim that mercury pollution is one of the greatest threats facing developing fetuses, infants, and young children. These experts believe that the subtle effects of mercury exposure include a reduced attention span, poor fine motor control, delayed language development, impaired memory, and difficulty with visual-spatial tasks such as drawing. Low levels of prenatal exposure can reduce intelligence, language development, memory, attention, and gross motor skills of offspring.[6] Larger exposures at crucial points in development can cause seizures, developmental delays, and mental retardation.[7]

☐ Lead: When young children are exposed to lead, attention deficits, hyperactivity, impulsive behavior, IQ deficits, reduced school performance, aggression, and delinquent behavior may result.[8] Such disorders are being seen with lead levels lower than the current safety threshold.[9] Studies have confirmed that blood lead levels greater than 10 μg/dL cause lowered intelligence, behavioral problems, and diminished school performance. A 2005 study determined that even lower lead levels are associated with intellectual deficits. Environmental lead exposure has been linked with an increased risk for numerous conditions and diseases that are prevalent in industrialized society, such as reading problems, school failure, delinquent behavior, hearing loss, tooth decay, miscarriages, kidney disease, and heart disease.[10]

Preliminary evidence suggests that lead exposure during early development may lead to schizophrenia later in life.

☐ Manganese: Several small studies have shown that children with manganese detected in hair samples have increasing rates of attention deficit hyperactivity disorder.[11] Manganese is often added to infant formula as a supplement and is naturally present in soy formula.

☐ PCBs: Exposure to PCBs in the womb can cause impaired learning, reduced intelligence, altered behavior, and hyperactivity as well as impaired reflexes and delays in developing motor skills.[12] PCBs are thought to exert their negative effects on the brain by interfering with thyroid hormone.

☐ Pesticides: Some pest control products affect the thyroid hormone and may contribute to abnormal brain development in children.

☐ Brominated Flame Retardants: These also affect brain development by interfering with thyroid hormone.

☐ Solvents: The toxic effects of alcohol on the developing fetus are well known. What is not well known is that other solvents, such as toluene, xylene, styrene, and trichloroethylene (TCE, may have similar effects. Women exposed to toluene while pregnant had children with deficits in learning, speech, and motor skills. Solvents are present in many consumer products, such as nail polish, glues, paints, resins, gasoline, and cleaning agents. The health effects of these products have not been adequately studied.

☐ Arsenic: A ten-fold increase in mental retardation was seen among children in a Japanese community who drank powdered milk contaminated with arsenic in 1955. Emotional disturbances, abnormal patterns on brain wave tests, and poor school records were also noted among the unfortunate children. Children may be exposed to arsenic through contaminated drinking water, food, and treated wood.[13]

If we continue to breed chemically stunted children, what toll will this have on society? Will future generations be subjected to the same tortuous feelings of failure that Chris endures? Will America and other contaminated industrial nations fail in the global marketplace because there is not enough talent or intelligence among the people?

Let's overcome this epidemic by having more compassion for those who are "slow" or less intelligent. They are not stupid; they are polluted. Let's focus our attention on the clean up and support those who we trust to protect us from harm. It is time for us to all work together to protect our children and our communities from toxins.

Chapter 10

*T*he Nightmare of Cancer

"The Lord giveth and the Lord taketh away, but He is no longer the only one to do so."

-Aldo Leopold

No One Is Immune

Cancer has touched the lives of many. It has stolen childhoods, ripped apart families, and devastated communities. My mother was busy raising five young children when she was diagnosed with melanoma. Because her own mother died when she was very young, my mother understood the suffering children endure when they are forced to live apart from their siblings.

Such was the fear in her heart when she called me into her bedroom, informed me of her illness, and made me promise that I would keep all of us children together if she did not defeat the cancer. And so at the age of nine, the burden of cancer entered my life.

I am certainly not alone. Cancer has become so commonplace that nearly one out of two Americans will be diagnosed with cancer at some time in their life.[1] Although the risk of contracting cancer increases with age, children are by no means excluded from its fury. One out of 600 American children will be diagnosed with cancer by the age of 10.[2] This number rises to 1 in 400 by the age of 15.[3]

What Causes Cancer?

Cancer develops when the inherent ability to regulate cell growth is impaired allowing abnormal cells to multiply out of control. Some people are born with a genetic susceptibility to developing cancer; however, genetics are only a small part of the cancer equation. A Scandinavian study in 2000 found that while inherited factors increase a person's susceptibility to most types of cancer, environmental factors are "overwhelming" contributors to its development.[4]

In essence, the expression of genetic information can be altered by environmental factors. If we wish to prevent cancer, we must be aware of the environmental factors that alter genes leading to uncontrolled cell growth. Let's explore some of the environmental toxins that have been linked to several of the more common or devastating forms of cancer.

The Canary of Cancers

A diagnosis of cancer strips the afflicted of their dignity, precious time, and former priorities. But when cancer strikes a child it is an especially heinous crime. Cancer in a child behaves in the same revolting manner as a pedophile—it steals the child's innocence. Once a child experiences excruciating pain, devastating treatments, immense grief, and the prospect of death, they no longer have the luxury of living the carefree life of a child. They can no longer be sheltered from the harsh realities and tragedies of life.

Such punishment these impossibly young victims must endure. And despite their struggle and will to survive, far too many little angels succumb to cancer, its treatments, or to infections that prey upon their weakened immune systems. Excluding accidental death, cancer is the number one killer of American children.[5] Unfortunately, that number continues to climb.

The incidence of cancer in American children under 10 years of age rose 37 percent between the early 1980s and the early 1990s.[6] Leukemia and brain tumors account for about one-half of childhood cancers.[7] Acute lymphocytic leukemia increased 27 percent between 1973 and 1990 and glioma, a type of brain cancer, increased 40 percent between 1973 and 1994.[8]

The World Trade Center (WTC) tragedy may have inadvertently shed some light on the link between environmental toxins and the escalating rate of cancer in young people. Just five years after the WTC rescue workers were exposed to the noxious chemicals in the dust, many were being diagnosed with leukemia and lymphoma. The reason for this perplexing correlation is that toxins don't just remain in the lungs once they have been inhaled. Rather, they are absorbed directly into the bloodstream where they have free access to genetic material, which many toxins are capable of altering or mutating. Once the blueprint has been changed in this manner, a variety of abnormalities may arise.

The reason that leukemia and lymphoma are among the first types of cancer to manifest after a toxic exposure is because they are cancers of the blood cells and the blood cells have a very short life span. They are constantly being manufactured and then disposed of as newer ones are made. This means that mutations are passed down through many generations of cells very quickly allowing problems like cancer to arise far more quickly in blood cells than in other, slower replicating, cell types.

When miners wanted to know if the air was too toxic to breathe within a mine shaft, they sent canaries in first. If the canaries died it was presumed unsafe for the miners to enter. Therefore, childhood cancer (such as leukemia and lymphoma) is the canary of cancers. The escalating rates of these cancers signal an unsafe environment and a strong probability that an epidemic of slower growing cancers is destined to emerge later in the lives of all who have shared this toxic environment.

If we wish to turn back the rising tide of cancer we need to reduce future exposures to the chemicals most strongly implicated. These include:

☐ Pesticides: Exposure increases the likelihood of leukemia and brain cancer.

☐ Solvents: A group of chemicals that dissolve other substances commonly used in industrial products, dry cleaning, auto repair, electronics, painting, printing, and furniture repair. Household uses include furniture stripping and hobbies such as painting. Adhesives may also contain solvents. Children may be exposed to solvents by residues brought home on parents' shoes or clothing. Examples of solvents include paint thinner, turpentine, benzene, and toluene.[9] Children can inhale the solvent perchloroethylene (Perc) in closets that contain dry-cleaned clothing. Communities with higher levels of air polluted by Perc, which is emitted from dry cleaning establishments, have higher levels of leukemia.

Cancer Cluster: The novel, *A Civil Action*, by John Harr was based on a real life cancer cluster in the small Massachusetts town of East Woburn. A group of unfortunate children developed leukemia after solvents contaminated their well water. Numerous other medical problems were commonplace in this community as well.[10] Another leukemia cluster in Dover Township, New Jersey, was linked to drinking water contaminated by solvents.[11]

☐ Petrochemicals: These are products of petroleum or natural gas that are used to form plastics, dyes, pesticides, etc. Occupational studies have shown a link between parents who have worked with petroleum products and increased leukemia rates in their children.

☐ Combustion Byproducts: Children who inhale diesel exhaust or polycyclic aromatic hydrocarbons (PAHs), found in tobacco smoke or wood smoke, are more likely to develop leukemia. Industrial plants and wastewater treatment facilities may also discharge PAHs into the water supply. Diesel fuel and exhaust, petroleum products, and PAHs have also been associated with childhood leukemia if their parents were exposed occupationally.

☐ Dioxins: These are some of the most toxic chemicals ever produced. Dioxin is formed as a byproduct during the production of petroleum, polyvinyl chloride, and pesticides and during the chlorine bleaching of paper and pulp. Dioxins are released into the air from waste incinerators, chemical accidents, as well as in accidental fires in buildings with vinyl siding, PVC plastics, or similar items. They are then released into the air and deposit on the soil where they enter the food chain and are ingested by humans. They accumulate in human breast milk.[12] Dioxins are known to cause childhood leukemia.

☐ Cured and Broiled Meats: Children who consume hotdogs at least once weekly are at greater risk of developing leukemia while those who eat hamburgers at least once weekly are more likely to develop brain tumors.[13]

Evidence has confirmed that acute leukemia in very young children is often initiated while still in the womb.[14] For example, the risk of brain cancer in children is greater when the mother is exposed to pesticides while pregnant than when the child is exposed after birth. Another example is that eating at least one hotdog per week while pregnant has been associated with childhood brain tumors.[15] For this reason, it is important to limit environmental exposures to potential carcinogens in parents prior to and during pregnancy as well as in children after they are born.

The Dirty Dozen: The Stockholm Convention is an international treaty that has targeted the "dirty dozen" chemicals for elimination because they are so detrimental to life and are not easily broken down, meaning that it may take generations to be rid of them. Dioxins are one of the dirty dozen.

Parentless Children

Aside from the heart-wrenching loss of a child, cancer has another tragic way of ripping apart families. It can take away a parent, leaving a child to endure a chronic aching loss. When my friend, Bobbie, shared the story of the loss of her mother with me, I realized that the pain doesn't go away once the child has grown.

Bobbie smiles as she remembers her mother's laugh, pretty smile, and soothing voice. She clings to these memories, which are all she has left of her mother. It is devastating for her to acknowledge that these memories are beginning to fade.

She pauses, unconsciously furrowing her brow, as she recounts the torment she felt on the eve of her wedding day knowing that her mother would not be present to share her joy. She then recalls the anguish she felt after giving birth to her first child. Unable to stifle the sound of her heartache, concerned nurses came running to her bedside as she wailed aloud over the injustice of her mother's untimely death. Her mother would never have the pleasure of knowing this beautiful baby she had just birthed. Bobbie breaks from her reverie, looks me in the eye, and concedes that this was certainly not the greatest agony she had endured.

With eyes lowered she haltingly recalls being torn from her younger sister who endured physical abuse at the hand of her stepmother for the remainder of her childhood. A child herself, she had remained silent, helpless, and ashamed.

This is the plight of a 12-year-old girl who lost her mother to breast cancer.

Such losses are no longer rare. What is claiming the lives of so many young mothers?

As a female cardiology physician assistant, I have attended several conferences entitled "Women and Heart Disease" or something similar. These lectures typically begin with an eye-opening slide depicting heart disease as the number one cause of death in women. The speaker then proceeds to make women feel foolish for fearing cancer when it is so obvious that they are more likely to die of heart disease. This message always left me feeling a little uneasy. After all, I believe in women's intuition. There must be a valid reason why so many women fear cancer rather than heart disease. So rather than trying to persuade women to alter their mindset, I decided to do a little research. And what I found is surprising.

Breast Cancer is the Leading Threat to Younger Women: This statement was found on the American Medical Women's Association website, "Coronary heart disease (CHD) is the leading cause of death for women aged 35 and older, killing six times as many women as breast cancer." This statement lumps all deaths over age 35 together, including the elderly. When you look at each age group individually the results are dramatically different. Breast cancer clearly exceeds the rate of death from heart disease in younger women.

Excluding unintentional injury, the number one cause of death in women between the ages of 5 and 64 is not heart disease, but malignant cancer.[16] In fact, 1 in 50 women will develop cancer by the time they are 39.[17]

These statistics clearly explain the fear that is rampant among Americans who are raising a family. Cancer, not heart disease, has stolen more mothers from their children, has forced more mothers to select another to raise their children in their absence, and has placed more children in homes devoid of love or in the path of abuse.

So why is there so much hype over heart disease? Perhaps there is too much to lose if we focus on an illness that is largely environmentally mediated. Those who fear heart disease worry about their cholesterol levels, blood pressure, blood sugar, and exposure to tobacco smoke, whereas those who fear cancer worry about what has contaminated their food, water, and air. From the standpoint of corporate polluters and their political enablers, it is beneficial to circumvent our concerns about toxic exposures and cancer by substituting the fear of an illness that is largely blamed on factors that require us to make lifestyle changes or take expensive medications.

A Women's Scourge

Breast cancer is the most common cancer diagnosed in American women, regardless of color. It causes the death of more women of child rearing age than any other cancer.[18] The number of women living with a diagnosis of cancer in 2002 was about one-half the number of children born in all of America that same year.[19]

The number of women diagnosed with breast cancer continues to rise, increasing by 43 percent between 1973 and 1998.[20] One in eight women now become victims.

A study of twins revealed that only 27 percent of breast cancer is a result of inherited genetic factors. Environmental causes account for the rest.[21]

The US National Toxicology Program has identified 42 chemicals as breast carcinogens according to results from animal studies. Internationally, 100 chemicals have been implicated. Many of these chemicals are commonly encountered in the form of auto exhaust, power plant releases, fossil fuel-burning processes, furniture finishes, dyes, solvents, natural estrogens and pharmaceutical estrogens (e.g. birth control or hormone replacement therapy). [22]

Exposure to ionizing radiation from x-rays, CAT scans, mammograms, and other medical studies is another established cause of breast cancer. [23]

Substances that mimic estrogen have been shown to promote breast cancer. These substances can leach out of plastic products and are also found in detergents, fuels, pesticides, personal care products, cosmetics, and even as inactive ingredients in many medications. Bisphenol A, found in commonly encountered plastic products, has been linked to abnormal development of the breast. Early life exposures may be especially important in the risk of developing breast cancer later in life.

Pesticides and solvents such as formaldehyde and benzene have also been linked to increased risk of breast cancer, particularly with the higher exposures seen in occupational settings.

Probable links to breast cancer include many pesticides and combustion by-products such as dioxins. Electromagnetic fields, chemicals in sunscreens, plasticizers, and growth hormone are possibly linked to breast cancer. Common sources of exposure to many of these breast carcinogens, and how to avoid them, are discussed in the next section.

What About Dads?

Men are more likely to be diagnosed with prostate cancer than any other cancer. It is second only to lung cancer in deaths due to cancer in men. Prostate cancer afflicts significantly more Black men than White men.[24]

Prostate cancer has been linked to substances such as pesticides, hydrocarbons, and combustion products. Men who are employed as firefighters, power plant operators, heavy equipment operators, or farm machine operators may encounter such chemicals and be at higher risk of developing prostate cancer. Metals such as arsenic and cadmium have been linked to prostate cancer as well.[25]

Hormone disruptors may lead to prostate cancer later in life if boys are exposed at critical times in their early development. For instance, even low levels of a chemical (bisphenol A) that leaches out of plastic have been shown to enlarge the prostate in animal studies.[26]

Animal fat, particularly from red meat, has also been linked to prostate cancer. This may be due to the production of carcinogenic chemicals from charring while cooking, the toxic chemicals stored in the animal fat, or characteristics of the meat itself.[27]

But I Don't Smoke

Lung cancer kills more people, regardless of gender, than any other cancer. It is more common in men than women and more common in Black men than White men. The incidence of lung cancer has increased considerably between the 1970s and the 2000s.[28]

Smoking and exposure to environmental tobacco smoke (formerly known as second-hand smoke) have been established as risk factors for lung cancer. This smoke contains nearly 5000 chemicals, 43 of them known carcinogens. The US CDC describes tobacco use as "the single most important preventable risk to human health in developed countries and an important cause of premature death worldwide." While tobacco smoke is a well known and important risk factor to the development of this most deadly of cancers, it is by no means the only risk factor.

Substantial evidence has linked petrochemicals and combustion byproducts, pesticides, silica, wood dusts, and asbestos to lung cancer.[29]

With every 10 microgram increase in invisible air pollution produced by coal burning power plants or diesel vehicles, there is an 8 percent increase in death from lung cancer.[30] In fact, one study showed that the risk of dying from lung cancer is the same for those who live with a smoker as for those who breathe polluted air.[31] The Journal of the National Cancer Institute reported in the 1960s that those residing in urban areas had double the chance of dying from lung cancer than those in rural areas—regardless of whether they smoked.[32]

Cancer Clusters

Determining the cause of disease clusters is difficult. Proving that they even exist is a chore as well. When communities notify public health officials of a cancer cluster, officials often determine that no cluster exists. They frequently refer to them as "The Boy Who Cried Wolf" cases.

Environmental experts argue that there are far more clusters than are admitted by officials at health departments or the Centers for Disease Control. In the case of the childhood leukemia cluster of Woburn, Massachusetts, it took intense media attention and litigation to force the department to re-analyze the data. Their findings were then reversed indicating a cluster of illness linked to an environmental cause.

Few disease clusters receive intense media attention or are successfully litigated; therefore, they are rarely linked to their cause. A few successes include: black lung disease caused by coal mining, a cancer of the lung called mesothelioma caused by asbestos, and cancer of the blood or liver resulting from the manufacture of polyvinyl chloride.

The burden of establishing proof of cause and effect in toxic exposures is enormously difficult. Such difficulty provides little opportunity for corporations who release toxic chemicals to be truly held accountable. It generally requires enormous exposure levels and previously extraordinarily rare diseases to link an environmental toxin to a disease. But this is not how it happens in real life.

We now know that miniscule amounts of toxins at crucial stages of development or over long-term exposure are capable of devastating outcomes. It is also true that chemical toxins are so pervasive in our environment and in our bodies that illnesses such as autism, cancer, and other chronic diseases have already escalated everywhere and are not rare enough for clusters to stand out. Rather than viewing the escalating disease rates as an obvious indication of an environmental problem, it obscures the picture. After all, a cluster is defined by the number of cases relative to other populations. The migration of chemicals to every corner of the world along with the soaring rates of chronic illnesses, cancer, and developmental diseases makes it nearly impossible for clusters to stand out.

Who is Winning?

Advances in medicine are directed at screening, diagnosing and treating rather than preventing this wretched disease, destroyer of families, and violator of innocence. The cancer establishment has successfully diverted our attention from the need for prevention by hosting a media campaign that proclaims we are "winning the war on cancer."

If we are winning the war, shouldn't fewer people be contracting cancer? This is certainly not the case. Between 1950 and 2001, cancer cases have increased dramatically.[33]

☐ Lung and bronchial cancer has increased 685 percent in women and 204 percent in men.

☐ Prostate cancer, myeloma, thyroid cancer, non-Hogkin's lymphoma, and liver cancer have all increased by over 200 percent.

☐ Kidney cancer, testicular cancer, and brain and other nervous system cancers have increased by over 100 percent.

☐ Breast cancer has increased by 90 percent in women and bladder cancer has increased by 97 percent.

These numbers are shocking and represent a far more serious problem in the US than previously suggested. And Americans are not alone. Cancer is an epidemic endured by all industrialized nations.

If more people are getting cancer, perhaps "winning" has been defined by cures. The term "cure" in the realm of cancer signifies that the victim has survived for more than five years from the time of diagnosis. A cure does not imply that the battle is over. A cure does not mean that the victim will not succumb to a relapse or cancer of another type later in life. Even with this forgiving definition, the cure rate is abysmally low. Only 50 percent of White victims survive, and the survival rate for Black victims is an appallingly low 38 percent.[34]

However, it is true that more children are defeating cancer. But have you seen what these "winners" have endured in order to be given a chance to live? The hope radiating from their eyes scarcely veils their pain in much the same way as their hats and scarves fail to disguise their hair loss and their hospital gowns inadequately conceal an assortment of wounds and tubes. These were once children. They were once able to run and play and laugh and torment their siblings. Now they are prisoners of the healthcare system. Is this what winning looks like?

> **Why Bother?** Cancer has ravaged so many communities that when it is suggested that a product be avoided because it has been implicated in causing cancer many people throw up their hands exclaiming, "Why bother? Everything causes cancer." While this may seem true today, it certainly hasn't always been the case. Cancer rates have climbed dramatically since the advent of the Industrial Revolution creating a deadly epidemic within a few generations. Previous generations certainly didn't believe "everything causes cancer," because in their generation everything did not cause cancer. This distinction should provide great hope. We don't have to endure this epidemic in future generations. If we dramatically reduce the production of toxic chemicals now, our children's children will not have to endure the pain of cancer to the extent that is seen today.

Sink or Swim

Cancer devastates more young American families than any other cause. Naturally, one would expect that the highest priority would be given to determining its causes and preventing them. However, the specific causes of childhood cancer remain obscure. Perhaps this is because the media hype has diverted our attention as well as the federal government's funding for research to other endeavors. Less than 3 percent of the 1995 federal government's research capabilities were devoted to this area.[35]

Funding research and programs that benefit heart disease at the expense of programs to prevent cancer prioritizes the causes of older Americans rather than young families. Why has our country chosen to place the elderly in the lifeboats while forcing the children and their young parents to sink or swim?

The limited resources that are allocated to this area are predominantly focused on genetic and lifestyle causes of cancer rather than on initiatives to reduce exposure to synthetic chemicals. Cancer is environmentally mediated, and therefore preventable. A marked increase in our federal government's research capabilities should be directed at studies to identify prevention strategies and for pollution prevention.[36] If attention were diverted to avoidance of toxic chemicals, cancer can, and shall, be prevented.

In the absence of protective legislation, the greatest hope for preserving families is to take matters into our own hands by learning how to limit our exposure to toxic chemicals. The next section provides the knowledge needed to do so.

*E*veryday Exposures and Problem Products

Everyday decisions, such as what to eat or drink, what type of medical or dental care to choose, or which products to use in and around our homes, play a major role in determining whether we will one day succumb to illness. Yet scant information is available to help us make sound choices. This section serves to increase awareness about the health hazards that may result from commonly encountered products and services and how to circumvent such threats whenever possible. The following is a wealth of frequently overlooked information that is crucial to our health and well-being.

Chapter 11

*F*rightening Food

"Tell me what you eat and I will tell you what you are."
─Jean-Anthelme Brillat-Savarin

Although wholesome foods contribute many of the nutrients we need to eliminate toxins and maintain health, food ingestion is also a major source of exposure to toxic substances. According to the National Cancer Institute, 35–50 percent of all cancers are caused by what we eat.

A nuclear technician once told me a surprising story. She recalls performing scans on cancer patients to see if malignant cells had spread to distant sites within the body. Interestingly, the imaging agent was always attached to glucose, a form of sugar, before it was injected into the patient's bloodstream. When I asked her why this was significant she replied, "Because the sugar carries the imaging agent directly to the cancer; the cancer feeds on it."

Sugar is not the only food that fuels disease. Foods that provoke inflammation, such as fried foods, trans fats (partially hydrogenated oils), and other processed foods, are capable of causing a host of medical problems. Yet reducing or eliminating sugar and other inflaming foods is no longer enough to ensure health. Much of our food supply has been stripped of its nutrients, tainted by chemicals, or contaminated by bacteria and other living things, before it reaches our tables. Such adulteration of our food supply has laid the groundwork for the epidemic of chronic disease that is our generation's legacy. In order to preserve or reclaim health we must learn how to avoid tainted food.

Food Additives

Additives are used to preserve, process, or cosmetically enhance food. As the use of food additives has dramatically increased, so have reports of intolerances and adverse health effects.[1] Artificial colorings are especially troubling and should be avoided whenever possible, particularly Blue 1, Blue 2, Green 3, Red 3, Yellow 6. Those who are allergic to aspirin should also avoid Yellow 5.[2]

The preservatives BHA, BHT, and propyl gallate prevent oils and foods containing oils from becoming rancid. The US Department of Health Services classifies BHA as "reasonably anticipated to be a human carcinogen" based on its ability to cause cancer in animals. Although the cancer connection is less clear with BHT and propyl gallate, it is wise to limit or avoid their ingestion whenever possible. Look for products that contain Vitamin E (tocopherol), which is a safer alternative for food preservation.[3]

Be on the Lookout for New Additives: While reviewing the ingredients in my former favorite junk food, peanut butter cups, I discovered an ingredient I hadn't seen before: TBHQ. A query to The Center for Science in the Public Interest informed me that TBHQ is structurally similar to BHA and BHT and that its safety has not been confirmed.

Nitrates (or nitrites) are often used to prevent lunchmeats, bacon, hotdogs, etc. from turning gray. When they enter the stomach, nitrates can form potent cancer-causing chemicals called nitrosamines. Pregnant women are strongly advised to avoid nitrates because they place unborn children at an increased risk of cancer. Eating at least one hotdog per week while pregnant has been associated with brain tumors in children.[4] Increased leukemia rates have also been seen in children who consume hotdogs and other cured meats regularly.

Although proper refrigeration/freezing of food would eliminate the need for nitrates, there are very few nitrate-free alternatives available. If you aren't ready to eliminate cured meats from your diet, the following suggestions may reduce your cancer risk:

  ☐ Substitute your current cured meats with those from Applegate Farms, which makes nitrate-free deli products.

  ☐ Add fresh tomatoes to a deli sandwich; choose a side dish of steamed or stir-fried broccoli or peppers; drink a glass of fresh-squeezed orange juice with your bacon at breakfast. All of these options add Vitamin C (ascorbic acid) to your meal, which decreases the formation of nitrosamines, thereby reducing the meat's ability to cause cancer.[5]

☐ Replace potato chips with a handful of almonds, hazelnuts, or sunflower seeds. These all contain a healthy dose of Vitamin E, which also prevents the conversion of dietary nitrates to cancer-causing nitrosamines.

What About Natural Flavors? While I was at a conference for professionals entitled, *Food as Medicine*, we were shown a slide that listed about 20 chemicals and asked to identify what the slide depicted. After a few moments of silence, the speaker replied, "natural strawberry flavoring." That is when I decided to avoid products that list artificial or natural flavorings in their ingredients. If it were a wholesome item it would be listed as an ingredient, not hidden in a generic term like "flavoring."

Potassium bromate is known to cause cancer in animals. In 1999, the Center for Science in the Public Interest petitioned the US FDA to ban potassium bromate, [6] but was unsuccessful. It is often added to bread and rolls in the US and Japan, but has been banned virtually everywhere else. It is rarely used in California because their stringent labeling laws may require a cancer warning on the label. If you find it difficult to locate preservative-free bread that is affordable, try baking your own. Here's a simple recipe that does not require a food processor, bread maker, or any expensive equipment:

1. Dissolve ½ tsp sugar in 3 cups of warm water. (The sugar is necessary to feed the yeast and the water can't be too hot or the yeast will die.)
2. Sprinkle a package of yeast (buy this in the grocery store; it is near the flour) over the water and let it sit for a while to proof. (Just place a moist cloth over the bowl and set it in a warm spot outside or in your kitchen. Five minutes should do the trick if it is warm enough. It will look sort of bubbly on top when it is ready.)
3. Add 1 tablespoon salt (I prefer sea salt) and about 4 cups of flour (white wheat, or a mixture of regular flour and whole grain flour will do, if you use only whole grain flour add some honey) and stir it up real good.
4. Just keep adding flour until the dough gets stiff. Then take it out of the bowl and knead it on a floured

surface. (Use your two hands and push the dough down and away from you, then give the dough a ¼ turn and repeat over and over until it is as smooth as a baby's bottom. This is a great form of stress relief and burns a few calories so consider your weekend bread baking session a wonderful alternative to yoga or light exercise and enjoy!) Keep adding flour as needed so it doesn't stick to everything.

     5.   Now just spread a little oil (Olive or Canola are my favorites) around a glass or stainless steel bowl and place the dough in it. (The bowl should be at least twice the size of the dough or divide the dough into separate smaller bowls.) Place a wet cloth over the bowl and set it someplace warm to let it rise until its double in size. (I usually put a piece of plastic wrap over one bowl and store it in the fridge for up to a few days for later use. The other bowl is set in the sun to rise for an hour or for the day, depending on my schedule.)

     6.   Knead the dough on a floured surface, briefly this time, and then shape into an oval loaf (like Italian or French bread) on an oiled baking sheet. (You can make rolls if you prefer.)

     7.   Place on the top shelf of the oven and bake at 450 degrees for 15 minutes or at 350 degrees for longer. (It is done when it sounds hollow when you tap the bottom with a spatula) Place a pan of water on the bottom shelf for better bread. (I forget sometimes too!)

     8.   Later in the week, when you are in a rush, you can use the remaining dough for more fresh bread by just shaping it on an oiled baking sheet, and placing it in the oven while it preheats (it will rise a little as the oven warms up). It also makes great pizza dough.

Avoiding Food Additives

If you are finding it increasingly difficult to go grocery shopping without a chemistry degree, you are not alone. One solution is to avoid the center aisles whenever possible and shop only the perimeter of the store. Limit your purchases to primarily organic produce, meat (if you eat it), beans, brown rice, nuts, and seeds. On the occasions that you desire packaged or processed foods, read each ingredient listed; if you are unsure what it is, avoid the product or look the ingredient up at **http://www.cspinet.org/reports/chemcuisine.htm.** This website is written for all to understand, with or without a science background.

The best way to avoid food additives is to avoid prepared foods. When it comes to healthy eating, there is simply no substitute for good, old fashioned home cooking. Although it can be difficult to find time to cook from scratch, the rewards are great. Try preparing meals on the weekends and storing them in glass containers in the refrigerator or freezer until needed.

A Healthier Place to Eat Out: I recently discovered that Panera Bread has an affordable grilled cheese children's meal that is made with their homemade, preservative-free bread and organic cheese. It is accompanied by organic yogurt and they sell organic juice boxes. Hooray!

Artificial Sweeteners

Aspartame (Equal, NutraSweet) is present in over 6,000 diet products including soft drinks, chewing gum, candy, desserts, and yogurt. It is also found in medications, particularly syrups and antibiotics for children. Hundreds of people worldwide consume aspartame, which has been maintained as safe by the US FDA despite a 1970s study in rats suggesting that aspartame causes brain tumors. A 2005 study confirmed the link between aspartame and cancer[7] and a 2007 study revealed that pregnant rats that were exposed to aspartame had offspring with higher rates of leukemia, lymphoma, and mammary (breast) cancer.[8] The cancer risk was evident at doses much less than the current acceptable daily intake.[9] It is advisable to avoid aspartame altogether, particularly in young children.

Saccharin and Acesulfame-K are other sweeteners that have been linked to cancer and should also be avoided. Saccharin (Sweet N Low) has been shown to cause cancer of the bladder, uterus, ovaries, skin, blood vessels, and other organs in animal studies. It can also increase the potency of other cancer-causing chemicals. The cancer warning that was once present on saccharin products has been removed due to commercial pressure. Acesulfame K is an artificial sweetener found in baked goods, chewing gum, gelatin desserts, and soft drinks. Animal studies suggest it might cause cancer and its breakdown product has been linked with thyroid problems in animal studies.[10]

Stevia (stevioside) is a natural sweetener obtained from a shrub in Brazil and Paraguay that is believed to be a safe alternative to synthetic sweeteners. Unfortunately, its safety is not yet confirmed. The Center for Science in the Public Interest believes that small quantities may be safe, but use should be limited until its safety can be established.

Irradiation

Irradiation of food has been touted as a major advance in protecting our food supply from bacteria and other infectious organisms. A massive amount of radiation is required to irradiate food: 10–100 million times the dose of a chest x-ray and up to 10 billion times stronger than the energy of a microwave oven.[11]

In order to irradiate food, a radiation facility utilizes enormous amounts of radioactive material leading to a tremendous increase in the amount of radioactive waste in the environment. The radioactive material used in food irradiation, cobalt-60, will remain radioactive for up to 100 years and will need to be continually replaced as it degrades requiring the need for expanding nuclear waste disposal capacity.

Cobalt-60 reminds me of when my mother was treated for melanoma. Her doctors implanted cobalt into her eye socket in order to destroy the cancer cells that were growing there. When my family went to visit her we were required to wear lead garments and limit our stay to several minutes so as not to be adversely effected by the radioactivity. This seems an unlikely candidate for processing food.

Yet the irradiation of food was established as safe and effective by the National Food Irradiation Program, which was formed by the US Army and the Atomic Energy Commission (now part of the US Department of Energy). Although there was opposition from consumer groups, the US Army and the Atomic Energy Commission sought and secured US FDA approval for the irradiation of several food-packaging materials in the 1960s. Since then it has been used to sterilize food for astronauts and to extend the shelf life and eliminate pathogens in uncooked meat, meat byproducts, fresh eggs, spices, and other foods.[12]

Some who oppose food irradiation claim that it is used to mask the unsanitary practices of the commercial food industry and to escalate commercial profits by extending shelf life at the expense of providing healthier food to consumers. Others question the validity of safety studies from vested interests such as the US Atomic Energy Commission, which was searching for a market for its surplus of radioactive materials after World War II.

Recent studies support those who doubted the safety of food irradiation. Irradiated food has been shown to promote cancer development and damage genetic material. Benzene and other toxins have also been found in larger amounts in irradiated foods. Animal studies have shown reduced survival rates and decreased immune system function as well.

Although proponents of irradiation claim it is insignificant, all food processing, including irradiation, causes a reduction in the nutrient quality of food. Food irradiation is particularly damaging to fat and fat-soluble vitamins. Omega-3-fatty acids, which are so beneficial to health, are damaged by irradiation as are some of the B vitamins and vitamin C.[13] It is just one more way of eroding the quality of food. There is simply no substitute for fresh, wholesome food with intact nutrients.

The 2002 Farm Bill included a provision that allowed the definition of pasteurization to include any process approved to improve food safety, including irradiation. This provision has further eroded the consumer's right to know what they are eating and feeding to their loved ones as irradiated food will no longer be labeled "irradiated;" rather it will simply say "pasteurized."[14]

> **School Lunches:** The Farm Bill of 2002 approved the use of irradiated meat for schools participating in the school lunch program.

Given the lack of appropriate labeling, the best way to insure that the food you purchase has not been irradiated is to purchase only organic food, particularly spices, meat, meat products, and eggs. Since 2001, the US Department of Agriculture's (USDA's) National Organic Program has prohibited ionizing radiation in the production and handling of organic food.[15]

If you cannot afford organic food, choose food from local farmers. Join the online Holistic Moms group (**www.holisticmoms.org**) to learn where your neighbors purchase their healthier food. Support the Consumers Union (**www.consumersunion.org**) or other advocacy groups to demand improved sanitation practices, healthy conditions for livestock, and proper hygiene in the commercial food industry. Such precautions would eliminate the need for irradiation in the first place.

Pesticides

The National Academy of Sciences and the Environmental Working Group have both reported that pesticides in food are significant enough to cause *immediate* health problems in children and some adults.[25] Diet is a major means of exposure to pesticides in children. Children who ate primarily a conventional diet had pesticide breakdown products in their urine that were six times higher than children who primarily ate organic foods.[16]

The best way to avoid pesticides is to purchase organic produce whenever possible. If cost is a factor, try limiting the most contaminated varieties of produce from your diet. These are listed in Chapter 21. Growing your own produce is a very economical way of avoiding pesticides. If space is limited, try growing herbs, greens such as lettuce or spinach, and other foods from a windowsill, indoors near a sunny window, or on a balcony.

Growth Hormone

Despite having been linked to cancer and banned in all 25 European Union nations as well as Japan, Australia, New Zealand, and Canada because of human health concerns, the artificial growth hormone known as rbGH or rBST was approved by the US FDA in 1993.

While Monsanto researchers continue to assure the public of its product's safety, evidence is mounting that it may not be. Cows injected with growth hormone have higher levels of insulin-like growth factor 1 (IGF-1), which is capable of making cancer cells grow rapidly. Monsanto claims that altering hormone levels in cows does not affect the hormone levels of the milk. But, the US FDA admits that the artificial hormones given to cows do increase concentrations of IGF-1 in the milk they produce. The IGF-1 in milk is not destroyed by pasteurization or stomach acid so it is capable of causing health problems for those who consume it.[17] A Harvard study revealed that men with elevated IGF-1 levels in their blood were four times more likely to get prostate cancer than the average man.[18] Another study showed that women under 50 with high levels of IGF-1 were seven times as likely to develop breast cancer. The researchers believe that IGF-1 may be a greater risk of breast cancer than other established non-genetic risk factors.[19] Reports have also linked IGF-1 with an increased risk of lung and colon cancer.[20]

Apparently consumers are not happy with the addition of artificial hormones into the cows that supply their milk. The hormone's introduction into the dairy supply has had the unintended effect of catapulting sales of organic products upward; organic milk sales doubled between 1996 and 1997.

The food industry is beginning to respond to consumer pressure. Starbucks has requested that all of its dairy suppliers avoid using growth hormone. Ben and Jerry's does not use products that have been exposed to growth hormones. The largest dairy processor in the US, Dean Foods, is converting some of its facilities to be hormone-free. Many grocery chains, such as Safeway and Publix, have converted their store-branded milk to hormone-free varieties. The number of dairies using growth hormone continues to drop. For instance, all milk produced in Oregon is now hormone-free.

As more and more consumers insist on hormone-free dairy, Monsanto is stepping-up its efforts to eliminate the consumers' right to know. They have already successfully petitioned the US FDA to include a disclaimer stating "No significant difference has been shown between milk derived from rBST-treated and non-rBST treated cows" on all products that are labeled as hormone-free.

Monsanto is now pressuring the US FDA to eliminate rBST-free labeling, requesting the Federal Trade Commission to investigate the advertising practices of hormone-free products, and urging the US FDA to send warning letters to hormone-free producers.[22]

The Organic Consumers Association, Cancer Prevention Coalition, and the Family Farm Defenders are fighting back. In February 2007 they filed a petition urging the US FDA to require cancer warning labels on all US milk produced with the artificial hormone. They also requested a moratorium on the hormone, citing it is an "imminent hazard."[23]

To locate a supplier of hormone-free dairy products near you, go to **www.organicconsumers.org**. A few nationwide suppliers of organic dairy products that pledge to be growth hormone free include: Alta Dena Organics, Horizon Organic Dairy, Morningland Dairy, Organic Valley, Stonyfield Farms, and Wisconsin Organics. Growth hormones are not administered to sheep or goats so dairy products from these animals are all hormone free.

Monsanto's actions have inspired the Millions Against Monsanto campaign. To join, go to **http://www.organicconsumers.org/monlink.cfm** or search for them on MySpace.

Antibiotics and Antifungals

Recently a campaign was launched to limit the overuse of antibiotics in healthcare, which is blamed for the emergence of drug-resistant bacteria, the so-called superbugs for which we have limited treatment options. But the truth of the matter is that of the 24 million doses of antibiotics used annually in the US, only 2 million are prescribed to people. The rest are used in animal feed. In reality, the emergence of superbugs may be a result of the overcrowding and other inhumane conditions that leads to disease-prone animals that require the prophylactic use of antibiotics.

When Did Grocery Shopping Begin to Require a PhD in Chemistry? About two years ago I glanced at the package of cheese that I was preparing to buy and was surprised by one of the ingredients. It contained natamycin. Although I was not yet fluent in the language of food ingredients, I knew from my medical training that "mycin" meant antifungal, which I presume was added to prolong its shelf-life. Because I had no desire to begin feeding my two-year-old antifungal medicine in the form of cheese, I went back to the aisle in search of an alternate brand. I became discouraged when I realized that every brand contained the medication. Without my knowledge a new ingredient had been slipped into a product I had been buying for years. This incident alerted me to the fact that I now have to read entire lists of ingredients every time I shop in order to catch such changes.

Rocket fuel

Food also becomes tainted when toxins are absorbed from contaminated soil and water. A recently identified source of contamination is rocket fuel (perchlorate), which has poisoned the Colorado River from Las Vegas to the Mexican border. Crops that are irrigated with water contaminated with rocket fuel may be more toxic than the water itself.

This contaminated stretch of river is the primary or sole source of irrigation water for farms in California, Arizona, and Nevada that grow the great majority of the lettuce sold in the US during winter months. Tests have shown that lettuce accumulates rocket fuel at over 100 times the concentration found in the water used to produce it. This means that eating lettuce irrigated with water contaminated with even low levels of rocket fuel results in exposure levels significantly higher than the US EPA's provisional "safety" level. Despite this data, the US EPA concluded in 2002 that foods do not contribute to rocket fuel accumulation in the human body. The data from subsequent industry-supported studies have mysteriously been lost.[24]

Unfortunately, water is used to grow organic as well as conventional produce, so consuming any vegetables grown in contaminated water may result in toxic exposures of rocket fuel. The safest course of action is to avoid lettuce grown in this region. Other produce may not accumulate rocket fuel to the same degree as lettuce. If you prefer to grow your own vegetables, but live in an area contaminated by rocket fuel, water edible plants with water from a reverse osmosis water purification system approved to remove perchlorate. (See Chapter 13 for information about choosing a water purification system.)

If your water quality has been compromised by rocket fuel, the best course of action is to log onto **www.ewg.org** and join the effort to keep contaminated crops from the market, compensate the victimized farmers, and clean up the mess.

Cookware

Nonstick cookware, such has DuPont's Teflon, contains a coating that has been associated with increased cancer risk, particularly of the liver and bladder; it has also been associated with birth defects in animals. When pans are heated above 500°F (260°C), the coating begins to decompose, releasing toxic fumes that have killed numerous pet birds and sickened people. The Environmental Working Group demonstrated that normal pans reach this temperature with normal stovetop use such as preheating on high for just two minutes.

The broad term for the chemicals in nonstick cookware is perfluorochemicals (PFCs). PFCs are also found in stain resistant products such as Scotchgard and Stainmaster and water-resistant products such as Gore-Tex. They are found in fast food take-out boxes, clothing, carpeting, etc. These persistent chemicals accumulate in the food chain and are not broken down in the environment. Traces have been found in 100 percent of newborns[25] and 96 percent of children tested in 23 US states.

Because DuPont was well aware of the health hazards of Teflon more than 20 years ago, but neglected to share the information with the public, they reached a settlement with the US FDA in 2005.[26] In 2006, the US EPA and the chemical industry agreed to a voluntarily phase-out of products containing PFCs.

Other Sources of Teflon in Your Kitchen: Be sure your oven is not lined with Teflon and that burners do not contain Teflon drip pans.

Aluminum cookware and aluminum foil may also pose a health threat. Leafy vegetables and acidic foods, such as tomato sauce absorb the most aluminum over time. Limit exposure to aluminum by placing a sheet of unbleached parchment paper between foil and food, replacing aluminum cookware with safer alternatives, and limiting the amount of time food is in contact with aluminum surfaces.

Anodized cookware is aluminum cookware that has been placed in an acidic solution in the presence of an electric current causing a layer of aluminum oxide to form on the surface. Anodization reduces leaching of aluminum from cookware into foods.

Stainless steel cookware may contain iron, nickel, or chromium. Corrosion-resistant nickel is unlikely to leach into food, even if it is acidic. Some people are allergic to nickel and should avoid such pans if it poses a problem. Small doses of chromium, as in the quantity obtained from cooking with stainless steel, are considered healthy.

Cast iron pans leach iron into its contents. Fortunately, iron is not a toxin; it is an essential mineral. However, people who suffer from hemochromatosis, a genetic disorder that predisposes to iron overload, should avoid food prepared with iron pans. Tomato sauce and other foods rich in Vitamin C (such as green leafy vegetables, which actually contain more Vitamin C than citrus fruit) should not be cooked in cast iron pans because the nutrient will be destroyed when it contacts the iron.

Do You Have Hemochromatosis? One million Americans are estimated to have hemochromatosis. Manifestations vary depending upon where the excess iron is deposited. If you have blood relatives with hemochromatosis or are suffering from fatigue, joint pain, stomach pain, heart disease, elevated liver enzymes, diabetes, or impotence, ask your doctor to order a simple blood test called a transferrin saturation test or a ferritin level. Regardless of a diagnosis of hemochromatosis, post-menopausal women and older men may wish to donate blood regularly to prevent the possibility of heart disease and other toxic effects of iron overload.

Ceramic cookware (pottery) is glazed to resist wear. Pigments from imported products may contain harmful lead or cadmium and should be used only for decorative purposes. Some glass and enamel cookware is also glazed and the same precautions should be undertaken.

Stainless-steel and lead-free ceramic, enamel, or glass cookware are good choices.

The Adulteration of Food in the 1800s: The need to control the adulteration of food and food products is not unique to modern times. In Bradford, England in 1858, about 20 people, including young children, died and more than 200 fell ill after consuming candy made with arsenic. The deadly candy was a peppermint lozenge made from sugar and gum. Because of the expense of sugar, it was common practice at the time to substitute "daft," a cheaper substance. Daft was a generic term for a variety of substances including plaster of Paris, powdered limestone, and sulphate of lime. In the case of the Bradford poisoning, the daft supplier was ill and the person he sent to retrieve the daft from the cellar accidentally retrieved arsenic. Hence, the arsenic was incorporated into the candy. The tragedy, known as the Bradford sweets poisoning, led to a public outcry and the eventual passage of the Pharmacy Act of 1868, as well as legislation regulating the adulteration of food.[27]

Chapter 12

Genetically Modified Food

"The current generation of GM crops is not safe...regulatory oversight is insufficient...industry-funded studies are incompetent by intention and design, and...public health would be served by the immediate withdrawal of these high-risk foods."
–Jeffrey Smith, Author of *Seeds of Deception* and *Genetic Roulette*

Because of the heated debate that is raging over the genetic modification of crops, an entire chapter is devoted to this relatively new form of food adulteration.

What is a Genetically Modified Organism (GMO)?

Genetic Engineering is the process of taking a gene that has perceived desirable qualities and inserting it into another species, called the host, that doesn't naturally carry a gene for that property. The new, and supposedly improved, organism becomes a genetically modified organism or GMO.

Getting the host to accept a foreign gene requires a "promoter," which is a section of genetic material from a virus or other organism that is capable of "infecting" the target organism with the new genetic information. The promoter forces the host to accept the new gene and carry out its orders.

The world's first genetically modified (GM) crops were grown in the US in 1996 and three-quarters of the world's GM crops are still grown in North America.[1]

GMOs and Hunger

According to public opinion polls, most people who support the cultivation of GM food do so because they believe these crops will benefit the 842 million undernourished people in the world. GM food is seen as a possible salvation for the millions of people who might otherwise suffer from malnutrition or succumb to starvation.[2]

But there is no shortage of food. According to the Food and Agricultural Organization of the United Nations, the global production of cereal alone is sufficient to meet the energy needs of the entire population if it were distributed appropriately. In other words, hunger is a result of inequitable distribution of food rather than insufficient supply. Between 1960 and 1999 the production of the most important food, animal feed, and fiber crops increased from 252 to 700 million tons. During this time of increased food production, the number of chronically undernourished people in sub-Saharan Africa more than doubled. Therefore, viewing GM food as a panacea for hunger is shortsighted and overlooks the fundamental reason for its existence: the distribution disparity.[3]

Besides, the production of GM food crops does not appear to be tackling the issue of hunger. Currently 85 percent of GM crops are herbicide-resistant soybeans, insect-resistant corn, and genetically altered cotton. Such crops are the backbone of agribusiness and the processed food industry, which is fueling the obesity epidemic and further undermining our health. Their cultivation does not nourish those in need; rather it benefits large commercial producers by reducing the cost of processed food production. Increased production of nutrient-rich crops that would benefit the hungry, such as pigeon peas, chickpeas, and pearl millet, is not being addressed by the genetic engineering of food.[4]

Are There Negative Consequences of Genetic Engineering?

There are several unnatural consequences of genetic engineering that have the potential to cause unprecedented harm. These include the following:[5]

- ☐ Once a gene is artificially inserted into the host it is passed down to all future generations and can even be transferred to other species.
- ☐ Normal genes have complex feedback systems that allow a gene to be turned on and off as needed. Because foreign genes are unnatural there are no feedback loops in place to control them; therefore, they cannot be turned off. Essentially, the foreign gene directs the formation of a foreign substance that the modified organism cannot regulate.
- ☐ The viral "promoter" may interfere with the way the host's normal genes function or impact the normal chemistry of the organism in unknown ways.
- ☐ The foreign gene physically disrupts normal function in the area where it is wedged.
- ☐ Because the foreign gene cannot be turned off, it

robs other essential metabolic processes of vital energy.

  □ GM crops are exceedingly difficult to contain. The altered DNA may be carried by pollen, the wind, or other means to contaminate unmodified crops nearby. The Union of Concerned Scientists found genetically engineered elements in 16 of 18 supposedly unmodified seed varieties tested. The cause of the contamination was unknown, but represents a threat to maintaining the integrity of unmodified crops. Such pollen can easily contaminate organic or non-genetically modified crops nearby.

  □ Nearly two-thirds of US genetically engineered crops such as corn, soy, and canola have been designed to withstand lethal doses of herbicides. A 1999 report found that farmers planting genetically engineered "Roundup Ready" soybeans used two to five times more herbicides than conventional soybean farmers. The dispersal of these foreign genes to other species has caused the emergence of "superweeds" that are difficult to eradicate and threaten local ecosystems and biodiversity.

  □ Pesticide-resistant GM crops may not even be very effective at what they were designed to do; pests are already building up resistance to the genetically engineered "pesticide plants."

How Do GM Crops Affect Humans?
The effect of GM crops on humans is largely unknown because they have only been recently introduced and adequate safety studies have not been performed. A group of US FDA scientists raised concerns that GM foods might promote allergies, new diseases, and nutritional problems; however, their concerns were dismissed. It appears the silenced scientists may have been correct. When GM soy was introduced to the European Union there was a 50 percent increase in allergic reactions to the product. Symptoms included irritable bowel syndrome, digestion problems, chronic fatigue, headaches, lethargy, acne, itching or burning skin, eczema, nausea, and headaches.

In August of 2003, more than 100 people living near a field planted with a variety of GM corn known as "Monsanto's Bt" became ill. Most of the sick were the vulnerable elderly or children. They complained of a whole host of symptoms including high fevers, coughing, weakness, skin irritation, headaches, dizziness, extreme stomach pain, persistent vomiting, and allergies. Residents complained that the field had a pungent odor similar to that of a pesticide.[6] As it turns out, their sense of smell was accurate. Bt corn is made by inserting a bacterium called Bacillus thuringiensis (Bt) into the host. This bacterium produces a toxin throughout the entire plant (including the edible portion) that renders the plant poisonous to insects. The pesticide scent mentioned by those in proximity to the GM corn field was emanating from the plants themselves, which were genetically modified to be "pesticide plants". About 25% of the US corn crop is now planted in Bt varieties.[7]

The toxin produced by Bt corn kills insects by destroying their stomach lining. Unfortunately, the effects of the Bt toxin are not limited to pests. The toxin leaches into the soil where it is capable of harming micro-organisms essential to maintaining the integrity of soil. Monarch butterflies and beneficial insects such as ladybirds and lacewings can be destroyed as well. Recent studies have confirmed that GM crops cause harm in other species as well; they have caused abnormal cell growth in the small intestines of mice; liver and kidney toxicity in rats;[9] decimation of herds of sheep and cows; sterilization of cows and bulls; and reproductive problems in pigs.

The toxin may even be harmful to humans. A man living near a Bt field was admitted to a hospital with a stomach ulcer; blood tests revealed that he had been exposed to the Bt bacterium. Although the underlying cause of the man's ulcer was not identified, it is certainly plausible that the toxin, which is designed to kill by destroying the stomach lining, may be to blame.

The gentleman with the ulcer was one of many sick residents near a Bt field who had traces of Bt toxin in blood samples obtained by Dr. Terje Traavik, a scientist from the Norwegian Institute of Gene Ecology.[8] But proponents of GM crops have dismissed accounts of illnesses such as these. They claim that the Bt toxin has never been associated with sickness. However, safety testing has not been required or conducted. When illnesses that may be related to the crops arise, they are swept under the rug. In this case, Dr. Traavik was chastised for creating unnecessary "panic." The extent of the health consequences of GM foods may not be recognizable for many years, perhaps generations, particularly if we continue to turn a blind eye to them.

Ominous Outlook: Tampering with the genetic properties of food may cause the human body to be unable to assimilate the altered substance into energy and nutrients that are essential for survival.

What is Terminator Technology?

Terminator Technology is the genetic modification of crops so that they produce sterile seeds. This ensures steady profits to the purveyor of seeds while preventing farmers from continuing the tradition of saving seed for the following growing season.[10]

What is BioPharming?

Biopharming is the process of genetically altering common crops to manufacture pharmaceutical products and industrial chemicals. Such crops have the potential for massive devastation because they are being grown in open-air fields where they may easily contaminate nearby food crops and are indistinguishable from unmodified plants. Corn is by far the most popular biopharm plant.

An example of a biopharm product is a potent abortion-inducing drug that is grown in tobacco. The virus used as the promoter is capable of infecting tomatoes, peppers, and other crops. If contaminated, unsuspecting consumers of these food crops may be at risk of aborting their unborn children. Despite the inherent danger of biopharming, over 300 open-air field trials have already been conducted in undisclosed locations across the US with a variety of pharmaceutical/chemical products.[11]

What Do the Experts Say?

☐ Hundreds of scientists are calling for a moratorium on all genetically engineered foods and are alerting governments worldwide of their hazards.

☐ The Alliance for Bio-Integrity organized a lawsuit that refutes the US FDA's claim that genetically engineered foods are safe and are hoping to reform the US FDA's policy on GM food.

☐ *The Lancet*, a respected peer-reviewed European medical journal, stated that there are "good reasons to believe that specific risks may exist" and that "governments should never have allowed these products into the food chain without insisting on rigorous testing for effects on health."[12]

☐ On February 5, 2001 the Royal Society of Canada issued a report declaring the presumption of no increased risk to be "scientifically unjustifiable." In the words of the *Toronto Star*: "The experts say this approach is fatally flawed and exposes Canadians to several potential health risks, including toxicity and allergic reactions."

94

The majority of US commercially grown soy, cotton, canola, corn, and Hawaiian papaya are currently genetically modified. A small amount of alfalfa, zucchini, and yellow squash as well as the Quest® brand of tobacco are also genetically modified. Personal care products such as shampoo, soap, detergents, and cosmetics may also contain GM ingredients.[13]

What You Can Do

Avoid processed foods that contain food additives such as soy flour, soy protein, soy lecithin, textured vegetable protein, cornmeal, corn syrup, dextrose, maltodextrin, fructose, citric acid, lactic acid, and vegetable oil. Purchase only organic corn, vegetable oils, meat, and dairy products.

Visit the Institute for Responsible Technology website at **http://www.responsibletechnology.org** and join the campaign for GM-free schools and communities. While you are there, download a sample letter to take to your favorite restaurants as you request that GM ingredients be removed from the menu.

Some companies have been unable to move forward with plans for biopharming due to lack of investment capital. Be sure your investment portfolio does not include companies that are engaged in biopharming or the genetic modification of crops. More information about socially responsible investing is provided in Chapter 23.

Chapter 13

Worrisome Water

"Wherever there is water there is life, and wherever there is life there is water...Water is not merely necessary for life; it is the essence of life."
-Beverly Rubik

One in five Americans drink water that violates federal health standards.[1] Between 1998 and 2003, nearly 2 billion people in the US were served tap water with enough pollutants to cause health problems.[2] Of the 260 contaminants detected in US tap water, more than half have no enforceable safety limits. In other words, public health officials are not protecting us from the majority of these chemicals even though they have known health consequences and millions of us drink them every day.[3]

Because they are unregulated, most water contaminants are not mentioned on the annual water quality report we receive from our local water utility. These unlisted chemicals are dangerous. Many have been linked to cancer, reproductive toxicity, developmental problems, and immune system damage. They include rocket fuel (perchlorate), a gasoline additive (MTBE); chemical by-products of water disinfection, plasticizers (phthalates), which are chemicals that are used in industrial and consumer products, pharmaceutical drugs, and fuel combustion byproducts. Currently, there are no limits to how much of these chemicals may be present in tap water.[4]

What Can You Do About It?
The first step to ensuring adequate water quality is to inquire about the quality of your drinking water. You can start by calling your local water utility to request a copy of its annual water quality report. Although the report is titled "the Consumer Confidence Report," remember that less than half of contaminants will be listed. The *Making Sense of Your Right to Know Report* can help you interpret the report and can be retrieved from **www.safe-drinking-water.org/rtk.html/**.[5]

96

To find out what unregulated chemicals may be present in your tap water, check out **http://www.ewg.org/tapwater/**.[6]

Chemicals that leach into the groundwater also end up in well water. If you drink from a well in an agricultural area, pesticides and nitrates are likely contaminants. Be sure to have the water tested periodically. Resources can be found at **www.wellowner.org.**

Once you have an idea of what is in your water, you will need to decide which contaminants pose the greatest threat to you and your family. This will enable you to choose the best course of action. Some information is listed below about several contaminants commonly encountered in our drinking water.

Rocket fuel

Rocket fuel (perchlorate) has been found in the breast milk of 100 percent of women who were tested. It is also in the water supply of at least 43 states. Over 20 million residents of California, Arizona, and Nevada drink water from the Colorado River or other sources known to be contaminated with rocket fuel.[7]

Rocket fuel interferes with thyroid hormone production in unborn children, which may lead to abnormal brain development. Small reductions in thyroid hormone levels during pregnancy have been linked to mental retardation, vision, hearing and speech abnormalities, reduced IQs, abnormal motor skills, and abnormal testicular development in offspring. Older children with abnormal thyroid levels may exhibit attention deficit disorder or poor motivation to learn. Lower levels of thyroid hormone can also cause depression, anxiety, unexplained weight gain, fatigue, and sexual apathy.[8]

How on earth did rocket fuel manage to get into the bodies of each and every one of us? Rocket fuel, which has been made, used or stored at more than 150 sites in 36 states, has contaminated the water or soil surrounding these sites. Unfortunately, such contamination has found its way into our nation's water supply. Crops irrigated with the contaminated water transfer the toxin to the food supply in far greater concentrations than the water itself. Rocket fuel has also been detected in nearly all samples of cow's milk tested in California.

Currently, the public is largely unprotected and unaware of the dangers of rocket fuel. Based on scientific studies that have shown significant health problems at extremely low exposure levels, the Environmental Working Group seeks a safety limit much lower than the one the US EPA is considering.[9]

Know Who's Funding Your Information Source: The Council on Water Quality website states that "Unnecessarily strict standards for rocket fuel could cause water shortages and cost taxpayers millions—with no public health benefits." This website is supported by the following defense contractors: Lockheed Martin, Aerojet, Tronox, and American Pacific Corporation.

Despite corporate media campaigns to disregard the threats of rocket fuel, Barbara Boxer, US Senator and Chairman of the Senate Committee on Environment and Public Works, is seeking protective measures. In January of 2007, she introduced a bill mandating that the US EPA promptly establish a health advisory and a drinking water standard for rocket fuel. She has also introduced a bill to require testing of drinking water for rocket fuel and public notification if the water is contaminated.

In the meantime, rocket fuel can be removed from your drinking water with the use of a reverse osmosis purification system.

Department of Defense: Approximately 1 million people may have been affected by water contaminated by dry-cleaning and industrial activities at the Camp Lejeune military base in North Carolina from 1957 to 1987. The water was polluted by a solvent, trichloroethylene (TCE), which was created by a waste disposal site on the base, as well as tetrachloroethylene (PCE), a dry-cleaning agent.

These are the same chemicals implicated in the real life leukemia cancer cluster in East Woburn, Massachusetts, which was recounted in Jonathan Harr's bestseller, "A Civil Action" and the blockbuster movie starring John Travolta that followed. Cancer, birth defects, and other health problems have been reported by those who drank the water polluted by the base. While the Camp Lejeune incident is believed to have exposed the largest number of people in history to such high levels of the chemicals, the pollutants have contaminated numerous neighborhoods surrounding other military bases and industrial sites across the nation.[10]

Organic Chemicals
Volatile Organic Compounds (VOCs) are a group of chemicals that evaporate, or volatilize, when exposed to air. They are widely used as cleaning agents, degreasers, and liquefying agents in fuels, polishes, cosmetics, drugs, dry cleaning solutions, pesticides, herbicides, petroleum products and industrial solvents. Although hundreds have been identified in drinking water, there are far more varieties of organic chemicals in use than are monitored. Some common VOCs are TCE, tetrachloroethylene (perchlorethylene, or "perc"), styrene, benzene, toluene, and xylene.
Wells located near industrial or commercial areas, gas stations, landfills, or railroad tracks, may be contaminated with VOCs. Local spills or dumping may also contribute to groundwater contamination. Drinking water in agricultural areas is frequently contaminated by pesticides and herbicides, which are also classified as VOCs. Areas with highly porous or "thin" soils and shallow depths to groundwater are most vulnerable to contamination because it is easier for the chemicals to leach into the water supply.
Some VOCs are known or suspected carcinogens. In high doses some may impair the nervous system or cardiovascular system. Little is known about the cumulative effects of low-dose exposure.
If you believe your drinking water may be contaminated by VOCs, go to **www.nsf.org** to find a carbon filtration system that is capable of removing these toxins from your drinking water. However, the best way to avoid drinking water contaminated by organic chemicals is to prevent their entrance into the water supply. Contact your local hazardous materials site to dispose of paint thinner, solvents, paint or similar products; never pour them on the ground or into a septic system. Also, report commercial or industrial spills immediately.

Pesticides and Herbicides
Pesticides and other chemicals have been estimated by the US Department of Agriculture to contaminate the drinking water of 50 million Americans. Another study discovered that the drinking water in two of three cities tested contained multiple pesticides at levels that often exceeded the US EPA threshold for safety.[11] Children appear to be particularly sensitive to these chemicals, which have been linked to a multitude of childhood cancers including leukemia, neuroblastoma, Wilms' tumor, sarcoma, non-Hodgkin's lymphoma, and cancers of the brain, colon, rectum, and testes.[12]

Because pesticides and herbicides are classified as VOCs, they are removed by the same carbon filtration systems that meet the standards for removing VOCs.

Chlorination and Disinfection Byproducts

Chlorine, chloramines, and chlorine dioxide are frequently added to public water supplies for disinfection purposes. Chemical disinfectants, such as chlorine are effective at killing disease-causing bacteria and viruses, but are incapable of penetrating the protective outer shell of parasites such as Giardia or cysts such as Cryptosporidium. When chemical disinfectants interact with organic matter in the water, potentially dangerous byproducts can form. Chloramines, which are formed by adding ammonia to chlorine, are less likely to react with organic matter in the water. Although they are a weaker disinfectant, they dramatically reduce the formation of toxic byproducts. Some water companies have replaced chlorine with their chloramine cousins to reduce the potential for health problems.

An alternate method of disinfection employs ozone to "superoxygenate" the water, thus killing many bacteria and viruses. However, microbes may reinfect the water during storage. For this reason, most water utilities combine ozonation with chemical disinfection processes.

If you have a commercial water source, it is likely that you have disinfection byproducts in your drinking water. These are easily removed with a carbon filtration device, such as the Brita or Pur pitchers or faucet attachments. Because the byproducts of chlorination are especially harmful when inhaled, be sure to purchase an additional filter for the shower and stand clear of the steam released when opening the dishwasher.

Sulfate

Water that smells like rotten eggs is likely to be contaminated with a form of sulfate called hydrogen sulfide. Sulfates are removed from drinking water with the use of reverse osmosis or distillation.

Nitrate

Nitrogen is essential to all life. It is present in the earth's atmosphere but must be restructured in order to be useful. Bacteria in the soil are capable of converting nitrogen to its usable form so that plants can use it for photosynthesis; thereby allowing them to grow. Most crops require large quantities of nitrogen for high yields.[13] Animals obtain the nitrogen they require to build proteins and genetic material by eating plants. The process of converting nitrogen into a usable organic form for all living things is called the nitrogen cycle.

Nitrates are formed as an intermediate step in the nitrogen cycle when microorganisms break down fertilizers, manures, decaying plants, or other organic matter. The addition of fertilizers and manures often results in the contamination of groundwater with nitrates that "runoff" the land. A safer method of replenishing the nitrogen level of soil is to improve the activity of microorganisms that convert nitrogen to its usable form or to plant legumes such as peas or beans in nutrient-poor soil. These crops naturally enrich the soil with nitrogen because the special bacteria that live in their roots are able to convert nitrogen to its usable form.

Although nitrate is considered harmless in moderate quantities, prolonged intake of high levels of nitrate is linked to stomach problems due to the formation of nitrosamines, which have also been shown to cause cancer in test animals.[15] Recall that children who eat hotdogs and other cured meats are exposed to these nitrosamines and have a higher incidence of leukemia than children who do not eat such foods.

Nitrates pose an additional threat to infants under the age of six months. This is because nitrates can be converted into nitrites by bacteria in their stomachs. (Older children and adults have stronger stomach acid, which inhibits these bacteria, making the conversion to nitrite less of an issue after six months of age.) Nitrite interferes with hemoglobin's ability to carry oxygen, which may result in Blue Baby Syndrome, brain damage, and death.[16] For this reason, it is especially important that infants not drink water contaminated with nitrate.

Blue Baby Syndrome: Doctors refer to Blue Baby Syndrome as methemoglobinemia. Pregnant women and those with reduced stomach acidity or a certain enzyme deficiency are also at higher risk of methemoglobinemia. The most obvious symptom of methemoglobinemia is a bluish discoloration of the skin, particularly around the eyes and mouth. Other symptoms include headache, dizziness, weakness, or difficulty breathing. Because it is a life-threatening condition, anyone with the above symptoms should proceed to the emergency room immediately for treatment.[17]

Reverse osmosis systems are effective at removing nitrates from drinking water.

MTBE

When lead was banned as an anti-knocking agent in gasoline in the US in 1979, many suppliers replaced it with MTBE. The additive gained popularity after the Clean Air Act of 1992 because it was promoted to reduce automobile emissions by helping gasoline burn more completely.[18]

Unfortunately, MTBE rapidly leaches into groundwater and is now known to have contaminated the drinking water of more than 40 million Americans. MTBE is released into the environment primarily through spills, leaks, pipe ruptures, improper transfers and overfilling.[19]

MTBE is classified by the US EPA as a possible human carcinogen. It also imparts a foul odor and taste to water, even at trace levels, rendering it unpotable. Many states have banned or significantly limited the use of MTBE in gasoline, and a nationwide ban is currently under consideration by Congress.[20]

Radon

Radon is a radioactive gas resulting from the decay of uranium. It is found in rocky terrain or soil that contains granite, shale, or phosphate and can seep into homes through the foundation or dissolve into water supplies. Agitation of the water by showering or washing releases radon into the air where the odorless, tasteless, and colorless substance can be inhaled. Radon is known to cause lung cancer. [21]

If indoor air levels of radon are elevated, radon testing of the water is essential. If the air level is low, water testing is not required. Increasing ventilation in bathrooms, laundry rooms, and kitchens will reduce the threat of radon while carbon filters will reduce its level in water.

If radon is detected in your home contact a professional about installing a system to remove it.

Arsenic

Arsenic, a metalloid, is a notorious poison that was frequently used as a murder weapon in the Middle Ages.[22]

What is a Metalloid? Elements with intermediate properties between metals and non-metals are called metalloids.

Because symptoms of arsenic poisoning closely resemble cholera, its use as a murder weapon frequently went undetected.[23]

Arsenic Hijacks Our Energy Source: ATP is the unit of energy used to fuel all processes of life in humans. The P stands for phosphate. Because arsenic closely resembles phosphate, it can bind where phosphate should in the formation of ATP, but is unable to function, rendering our energy currency useless.

Although most arsenic exposure is due to the use of "pressurized wood" in decks, playgrounds, and picnic tables, as well as from arsenic-containing pesticides and mining practices,[24] more than 60 million people in the United States, particularly residents of parts of Michigan, Wisconsin, Minnesota, and the Dakotas, have dangerous levels of arsenic in their drinking water.[25]

Arsenic is strongly associated with lung and skin cancer in humans.[26] It has also been linked to bladder, kidney, liver, prostate, and throat cancer. High levels of arsenic exposure in a short time can cause death. Anemia, skin lesions, and burning, tingling, or numbness of the extremities are classic symptoms of chronic arsenic toxicity. Chronic arsenic ingestion may also cause cramping, diarrhea, anemia, high blood pressure, heart rhythm problems, heart failure, and impairment of the immune system. Arsenic can cross the placenta causing low birth weights, miscarriages, and other problems to the developing fetus.[27] It has also been found to limit the intelligence and growth of children.[28]

See the table at the end of this chapter to learn how to remove arsenic from your drinking water.

Chromium

Chromium poisoning was popularized by the 2000 movie, *Erin Brockovich*, which was based on the real-life contamination of the groundwater in Hinkley, California, with hexavalent chromium, or chromium 6. Residents of the town suffered from a myriad of health problems including elevated cancer rates.

In order to evade liability and expensive clean-up efforts, the industrial polluter (PG&E) tried to create scientific uncertainty by hiring scientists to reverse the findings of a study that showed drinking water contaminated with chromium 6 caused cancer. The fraudulent study was successfully placed in the *Journal of Occupational and Environmental Medicine* in 1997 without disclosing that PG&E had paid for it.[29] The study has since been retracted and a 2007 study by the National Toxicology Program concluded chromium 6 does cause cancer in laboratory animals when it is consumed in drinking water.[30]

Chromium 6 is removed from drinking water by reverse osmosis systems.

Lead

Lead is a heavy metal with potent nervous system toxicity, particularly to the developing brains and nervous systems of the unborn and very young children. Exposure during early development can cause permanent learning disabilities and hyperactive behavior. Long-term exposure to even low levels of lead can cause more subtle defects as well as high blood pressure, anemia, and nerve damage. Higher-level exposures may result in severe brain damage or death.

Lead contamination in drinking water usually results from lead pipes, lead solder joints, or brass faucets in homes or facilities built before its use was banned in 1986.

If lead is a problem in your community's drinking water, corrosion control measures should be enacted to reduce leaching of lead into water. For further protection from lead, let the water that has been sitting in the pipes overnight run out of the tap (about one minute) before using it in the morning. Because hot water tends to dissolve more lead from pipes, use only cold water to cook with or consume. For private wells, consider purchasing a calcite filter to reduce the acidity of the water thereby limiting corrosion.

Reverse osmosis, distillation, and ion-exchange filters are all capable of removing lead. Drinking bottled water is another solution, but one that is typically more costly to the pocketbook and environment.

Microorganisms

Microorganisms that are capable of causing disease are called pathogens. These include bacteria, viruses, parasites, etc. Historically, bacteria in water caused epidemics such as cholera and typhoid fever. Public water utilities in developed countries are now largely successful at eliminating such pathogens from the water. To avoid recurrences of these deadly diseases, the public is instructed to boil the water they consume or cook with in the event that a natural disaster or accident disables water treatment plants.

E coli is a bacterium that is transmitted through feces and often enters the water supply. It is regulated by the US EPA and disease outbreaks from water sources are rare. More troublesome pathogens are those that form cysts, such as cryptosporidia and giardia, which are resistant to typical disinfection processes. Both of these pathogens cause diarrhea often accompanied by nausea, abdominal cramping, and a low-grade fever, lasting a week or two; however, in those with compromised immune systems infection is more serious and potentially fatal. The US EPA admits that even properly functioning water treatment plants cannot guarantee that the water will be free of these extremely prevalent pathogens.[32]

The presence of giardia in virtually all surface waters is the reason it is no longer advisable to drink water from apparently clean streams and lakes. Once a person or pet is infected with giardia, they can transmit it directly to others as has been seen in daycare centers. This is why it is important to wash hands after changing diapers and using the restroom.

Boiling water for one minute at sea level and up to five minutes at higher elevations will kill giardia as well as other microorganisms. Iodine tablets are also useful to eliminate the threat of giardia from drinking water while camping or backpacking. Some filters marketed for this purpose may be ineffective at removing tiny giardia cysts.

To prevent others from becoming infected, always bury feces, human and pet, eight inches deep and at least 100 feet away from natural waters.

Tips for Safer Drinking Water

The contaminants listed above are just a small sampling of the thousands of chemicals that may be present in your drinking water. Given the rampant contamination of drinking water, it is extremely likely that you will discover you have poor water quality. Fortunately there are options for obtaining safer drinking water. If you have the luxury of affording safer drinking water please consider advocating for those who cannot afford to provide healthy water to their children. Go to **http://www.safe-drinking-water.org/** and join the Campaign for Safe and Affordable Drinking Water or seek out a struggling single mom or other less-fortunate family for whom you can provide a water treatment system. Several water treatment options are discussed below.

Boiling Water

Boiling water for one minute results in disinfection of water by killing most harmful infectious agents, but does not remove chemical toxins. Therefore, the decision of whether to boil water is based on the likely contaminants in the water and individual health concerns. For example, newborns are more susceptible to

105

the toxic effects of lead and nitrates than to infectious agents. Both nitrates and lead are concentrated in boiled water resulting in higher doses of these toxins.

For this reason, parents are no longer encouraged to boil water for the preparation of formula. This makes it a profound social injustice that poor children often have no other treatment option. Please join the crusade to make healthy drinking water available to all children.

People with weak immune systems should boil the water they ingest, brush their teeth with, or cook with as they are more susceptible to infectious agents.[33] Otherwise, boiling water should be reserved for emergencies when the need to eliminate the threat of bacteria arises.

Home Filtration Systems

There are several types of home filtration systems; activated carbon (charcoal) and ceramic are commonly used. Activated carbon filters are relatively inexpensive and convenient to use and install. They are relatively effective at improving taste and odor of municipal water as well as removing chlorination products. (Well water often requires specialized pre-filtration to remove sulfur or iron in order to improve its taste.)

Not all carbon filters are effective at removing VOCs, asbestos, giardia cysts, and heavy metals such as arsenic, copper and lead. If these contaminants are a concern, look for a filter that is certified for their removal. (Search **www.nsf.org** for a filter that meets the standards for their removal.) Carbon filters do not provide protection from rocket fuel, nitrates, sodium, or fluoride.

Ceramic filters are useful for removing bacteria, asbestos, and cysts, but are ineffective in reducing VOCs, byproducts of chemical disinfection, such as trihalomethanes, and heavy metals, such as mercury or lead. Ceramic filters can be combined with carbon filters to cover both bacterial contaminants, which ceramic filters are more effective at removing, and organic chemicals, which are dealt with better by certain carbon filters.

Filtration will not remove beneficial minerals from the water nor will it affect its alkalinity. Choose a filter that is certified by NSF International (**www.nsf.org**) to remove the contaminants of greatest concern in your water.[34]

Because inhalation of chlorinated products and other volatile chemicals is detrimental to health, consider employing a filter for the bath or showerhead as well.

Reverse Osmosis (RO)

This method of water filtration can remove fluoride, many bacteria, viruses and cysts, sodium, asbestos, and heavy metals such as arsenic, lead, mercury, cadmium, and aluminum. Some systems remove nitrates and chlorides while others do not. If you are going to undergo the expense of having a reverse osmosis system installed, be sure it comes complete with a carbon filter to insure the removal of additional toxic substances, such as VOCs.

Reverse osmosis is particularly useful in fluoridated areas or in wells contaminated with nitrates. If water is contaminated with microorganisms, ultraviolet treatment should be added.

The following are several drawbacks to reverse osmosis:

☐ It requires high water pressure.

☐ It can take a long time to process small amounts of water.

☐ A large quantity of source water is wasted by flushing away contaminants.

☐ The treated water is devoid of beneficial minerals such as calcium, magnesium, potassium, and sodium. (Mineral supplements may be required to prevent health problems.)

Distillation

Distillation boils the water, catches the resulting steam, and condenses the steam on a cold surface (a condenser). Nitrates and other minerals remain behind in the boiling tank. Distillation will commonly remove 99 percent of all bacteria, chlorine, arsenic, aluminum, pesticides/herbicides, lead, copper, other heavy metals, sodium, nitrates, and industrial solvents.

Volatile organic compounds are not effectively reduced by distillation alone. Therefore a final "post" filter of carbon is used to remove these contaminants. Thus, distillation followed by carbon filtration gives a very pure form of water. Drinking distilled water can dissolve some kidney or gallstones.

Disadvantages to distillation include the following:

☐ It requires a significant amount of electricity.

☐ It takes a long time to produce water.

☐ It requires significant maintenance.

☐ Water-cooled units waste 7–14 gallons of water per gallon (air-cooled distillers do not).

☐ Treated water is devoid of all minerals, including healthy minerals.

☐ The resultant water is acidic.

Ultraviolet Light
Ultraviolet light (UV) can be used to kill bacteria and viruses without the addition of chemicals to the water. To be effective, all of the water must be exposed to the light from the UV lamp. UV light is ineffective in reducing cryptosporidium and does not remove chemicals, solvents or heavy metals. It is usually used in combination with other purification techniques.

Water Softeners
The hardness of water relates to the amount of minerals that are present, most commonly calcium and magnesium. The more minerals that are present, the harder the water. While soft water contains very little calcium, magnesium or iron, it may contain sodium. Soft water is often preferred because it allows detergents and cleansers to lather more easily. It also eliminates mineral deposits in tubs, toilets, etc. Some people use water softeners to remove calcium and magnesium by exchanging them for sodium. The process is called an ion-exchange.

Unfortunately, there is a price paid for this "cleaner" water. Some of the drawbacks to soft water are listed below:

☐ It is devoid of healthy essential minerals.

☐ It is more acidic and therefore facilitates the leaching of lead, cadmium, and other toxins from the pipes into the water.

☐ The addition of high levels of sodium may compromise health: soft water has been associated with a higher incidence of heart disease, high blood pressure, and strokes.

☐ The tank must be periodically maintained by flushing it with sodium chloride (salt) to recharge it. (Automatic rechargers eliminate this chore, but you need to remember to keep the sodium storage container filled.)

☐ It has not been purified and will retain contaminants present in the source water.

Water Ionizers
A water ionizer is usually connected to the kitchen tap and works by filtering the water first to remove contaminants followed by electrolysis or ionization. Running tap water over positive and negative electrodes causes water particles to split, becoming ionized. The water is divided into two separate streams. One is alkaline for drinking. The other is acidic and can be used for cleaning.

Ions are electrically alive. The ions in the alkaline water will seek out acids to bind with in order to return to a stable, neutral charge. According to proponents of ionized water, this means that it is capable of neutralizing acidic waste products in the body, thereby preventing them from oxidizing, or rusting the inside of the body, which would lead to a host of illnesses. In other words, alkaline water is considered a potent antioxidant. Because of the tremendous number of health conditions reported to benefit from alkaline water, the water ionizer was reportedly approved as a medical device in the 1960s by the Japanese Ministry of Health, although I cannot find a reference to confirm this. For more information about water ionizers, go to **www.waterionizer.org** or **www.gobeyondorganic.com.**

Bottled Water

Current lax regulations allow industry to reap enormous profits while failing to clean up the messes they leave behind. This has contributed to 45 percent of lakes and 39 percent of streams and rivers being described as unsafe for drinking, fishing, and sometimes even swimming.[35]

Even when decontamination efforts are undertaken, they are frequently insufficient. One study revealed that conventional treatment techniques remove less than 20 percent of some contaminants.[36] As the public has become aware of the poor quality of drinking water, many have switched to drinking bottled water. Yet, bottled water is not always superior to tap water.

The National Resources Defense Council (NRDC), the most comprehensive publicly available independent testing of US bottled water in the US, conducted a study in 1999, which revealed the following sobering facts about the bottled water they tested:[37]

☐ One-third violated a state water quality standard or exceeded microbiological-purity guidelines.

☐ One-fifth contained VOCs or chemicals used in manufacturing plastic such as plasticizers (phthalates) or styrene.

☐ Many contained arsenic, nitrates, or other contaminants.

The NRDC concluded that, "there is no assurance that bottled water is any safer than tap water."[38] Moreover, they warn that as more consumers shift to bottled water, less funding may be made available to protect tap water, which the poor would remain dependent upon.[39] This would create a serious social injustice. Another concern about bottled water is that the plastic may leach

109

hormone disruptors into the water, which are passed on to the consumer.

The US Conference of Mayors recently adopted a resolution to use tap water rather than bottled water. Their reasoning included cost, the great distance the bottles must travel from their source and its inherent pollution, the millions of barrels of oil required to manufacture the bottles, and the enormous burden on landfills where water bottles have become "one of the fastest growing sources of municipal waste."[40]

When the environmental costs of packaging and distributing bottled water are factored into the bottled versus tap water equation, tap water prevails. Fixing our tap water so that it is safe and healthy for all is the only acceptable, socially equitable, long-term solution to our water quality crisis. In the meantime, selecting an individualized home purification process based on your specific contaminants is a good approach. If you still choose to consume bottled water, purchase it from a reputable company. Ask the company where the source of the water is located and how the water is treated, then request documentation to verify their claims.[41] Choose a supplier that has been approved by NSF International, which makes unannounced inspections. Go to **www.nsf.org** to select a brand.

The Canadian Bottled Water Association also provides a list of brands that meet their health and safety standards on their website, **www.cbwa-bottledwater.org**. The European Union has stronger standards to protect their bottled water than the US. They explicitly ban all pathogens and require natural mineral water bottles to label its source and composition.

Unregulated water: The lax drinking water safety standards provided by the US FDA do not apply to bottled water that is sold within the same state as its source. Such water is not regulated at all.

How to Select a Water Filtration Device

Step 1: Before purchasing a water filtration product, obtain a copy of the Consumer Confidence Report from your local water utility. Also check out **http://www.ewg.org/tapwater/** to identify which unregulated chemicals may be present in your water supply. If you drink from a private well, check out **http://www.ntllabs.com/homeowner/index.html** or

www.wellowner.org to find an independent testing lab. Your local health department may also have information about contaminants commonly found in your area.

    Step 2: Look up the standard for each of your top chemical concerns on the Contaminant Guide of the NSF website by going to **www.nsf.org,** then clicking on Consumer>Drinking Water> Contaminant Guide. Products that have this standard listed on their packaging will be most effective at reducing that particular contaminant.

    Step 3: Search the Product Guide to find a product that indicates it meets each of the standards you require based on the Contaminant Guide. To reach this page, simply click on the Search for Certified Products links on the menu to the left of the Contaminant Guide page.

    Step 4: Purchase the unit that most effectively meets your needs.

    Need Help? You can reach NSF in the US at 1-877-867-3435 if you require assistance.

How to Eliminate Common Drinking Water Contaminants

Contaminant	Examples	Elimination Strategy
Rocket fuel	Perchlorate	Reverse osmosis
VOCs	Benzene, styrene, THM, TCE, lindane, many others	*Filtration (carbon/charcoal)
Pesticide or herbicide residues	Alachlor, PCBs	Same as for VOCs
Chlorine or disinfection byproducts		Same as for VOCs
Sulfates	Hydrogen sulfide	Reverse osmosis or Distillation may be effective
Nitrate/Nitrite		Reverse osmosis
Radioactive elements	Uranium/radon	Reverse osmosis, Distillation, or Anion exchange resins may be effective
Arsenic	Pentavalent (arsenic 5 or arsenate) Trivalent (arsenic 3 or arsenite)	Pentavalent: reverse osmosis or distillation Trivalent: distillation or chlorinate to convert to pentavalent then use reverse osmosis.
Chromium	Chromium-6, Chromium-3	Reverse osmosis Distillation
Heavy metals	Mercury, lead	Filtration (carbon/charcoal) reverse osmosis, distillation
Parasites and cysts	Cryptosporidium, giardia Entamoeba and toxoplasma	Filtration (carbon/charcoal) Reverse osmosis
Fluoride		Reverse osmosis, distillation

This table is derived from information available at **www.nsf.org**
*Although the chart may list a strategy as capable of removing a particular contaminant, not all devices are equally effective. For example, some carbon filters remove VOCs while others do not. Reverse osmosis systems typically come with a carbon filtration filter, allowing more contaminants to be eliminated.

Chapter 14

The Fluoride Controversy

"I am appalled at the prospect of using water as a vehicle for drugs. Fluoride is a corrosive poison that will produce serious effects on a long-range basis. Any attempt to use water this way is deplorable."
- Dr. Charles Gordon Heyd, Past President of the American Medical Association.

What is Fluoride?
Fluoride is an ion, a charged particle that seeks to bind to oppositely charged particles for stability. This means that fluoride is a generic term for different chemicals depending upon the substance to which the fluoride ion has become bound. Some people say that fluoride is a naturally occurring element essential for healthy teeth. Others say it is an industrial byproduct capable of causing serious health problems.

Why is Fluoride Added to US Drinking Water?
North American water systems have added fluoride to their water supplies since 1945 to help prevent tooth decay. The fluoridation of drinking water is endorsed by the American Dental Association and the US Public Health Service. In 2000, the US Centers for Disease Control and Prevention (CDC) estimated that two-thirds of residents using community water systems, or 162 million people, had access to fluoridated tap water. That number continues to grow.[1]

Do Other Nations Fluoridate Their Drinking Water?
Nearly all of the European Union has denounced the fluoridation of drinking water. However, the English Parliament passed the Water Act in 2003 to allow water authorities to add fluoride to the public drinking water if health agencies request it, an action that has sparked strong opposition.

Does Fluoride Really Benefit Teeth?
Although fluoride is added to water supplies with the intent

113

to reduce tooth decay, the cities that have the largest percentage of water treated with fluoride are often the cities with the worst cavity rates. The US states with the highest rate of tooth loss are Kentucky and West Virginia, which both have very high rates of fluoridation. Conversely, Africa, which has the lowest rates of both dental care and fluoridation in the world, also has the lowest cavity rate in the world.[2]

Preserving Teeth or Worsening Health? Now that sugar consumption is increasing in Africa, the World Health Organization believes that Africa needs fluoridation to prevent future increases in its cavity rate.[3]

As it turns out, numerous studies indicate that fluoride does not prevent cavities. Most recent dental surveys have found no relevant differences in tooth decay rates between fluoridated and unfluoridated communities.[4] In fact, lower rates of cavities were observed in La Salud, Cuba, and British Columbia, Canada after water fluoridation ceased.[5] Tooth decay has declined globally, regardless of, or in spite of, community fluoridation status.

It is now known that fluoride delays the emergence of teeth in children, thus postponing the time until cavities develop. In other words, fluoride doesn't prevent cavities, it merely postpones their occurrence.[6]

What are the Health Consequences Associated with Water Fluoridation?

According to a 2005 US CDC study, 37 percent of American children have some form of dental fluorosis, up 9 percent from 20 years ago. Higher rates of fluorosis are seen in African Americans than Caucasian Americans.[7]

Dental fluorosis is the appearance of white spots, mottling, yellowing, or even brownish discoloration of the teeth. Fluorosis results from fluoride exposure before the age of 5 or 6; it cannot occur once the tooth has erupted into the mouth.[8] It is more common in children consuming drinking water with more than 1 ppm of fluoride and in those with a poor intake of calcium. Proponents of water fluoridation claim that dental fluorosis is merely an aesthetic problem, and therefore is acceptable collateral damage in the fight against tooth decay. But fluorosis weakens the teeth and the condition of the teeth is an indicator of the condition of the bone.

How Fluoride Affects Bone Cells: Normally, bone contains two types of cells with opposing jobs. The osteoblasts lay down new bone while the osteoclasts clear away the old. This process maintains the structural integrity of bones. Fluoride inhibits the cells that clear away the old bone, resulting in abnormal bone structure or uncontrolled bone growth.

Fluoride and Cancer

Because cancer is a result of uncontrolled cell growth, the increased rate of bone cancer (osteosarcoma) among children drinking fluoridated water should come as no surprise.

Although fluoridation increases the density of the bone, it does not result in stronger bones. Rather, it makes the bones more brittle and predisposes them to increased fracture rates, such as stress fractures in young people or hip fractures in seniors. Studies have found increasing rates of both with exposure to fluoridated water.[9]

The WHO warns that drinking as little as two liters of fluoridated water can lead to arthritis-like symptoms, which is the earliest manifestation of fluorosis within the bones. Severe skeletal fluorosis is a crippling bone disease. Cattle who suffer from this condition have been seen crawling on their bellies or grazing on their knees because of their inability to stand or walk.

Fluoride also wreaks havoc upon the brain. A large body of evidence has linked fluoride exposure to brain damage, such as impaired thinking and memory as well as fatigue and generally feeling poorly.[10] Chinese studies reveal that children who get more fluoride have lower IQs.[11] Children with fluorosis of the teeth are at greatest risk of brain impairment because fluorosis is an indicator of fluoride toxicity.[12]

Caution for Pregnant Women: Fluoride begins accumulating in brain tissue before birth.[13]

Additional toxicities of fluoride include:
- ☐ Liver and kidney damage[14]
- ☐ Earlier onset of sexual maturity[15]
- ☐ Cancer, especially of the bone[16]
- ☐ Increase in the number of Down's syndrome babies

born to younger mothers[17]
  □ Hormone disruption[18]
  □ Thyroid dysfunction [19]
  □ Increased blood sugar and worsening of diabetes[20]
  □ Stomach upset[21]
  □ May weaken the immune system because immune
system cells are made in the bone[22]
  □ Possible increase in Alzheimer's disease.[23]

Who Said Fluoride Was Safe?
     Fluoride is a byproduct of the pesticide, fertilizer, and
aluminum industries. It was also essential to the production of the
atomic bomb. In 1943, while the E.I. du Pont du Nemours
Company was producing millions of pounds of fluoride for this
purpose, an accidental release exposed the surrounding
community to toxic fluoride gas. The New Jersey farms downwind
began to report severe damage to their crops, death of their
poultry, sickened horses, and cattle that could no longer stand,
graze, or reproduce. Many residents complained of vomiting all
night. When the farmers filed suit, the US government worried that
many similar lawsuits might follow, thus impeding the bomb
program's ability to use fluoride. To prevent this perceived
catastrophic blow to national security, the US government began
conducting studies to prove the safety of fluoride. These safety
studies were marred by secrecy and the strong intent for a positive
outcome.

Where Does the Fluoride Come From?
     Once communities began filing lawsuits against industries
that were releasing fluoride gases into the atmosphere, pollution
control measures were begun. Fluoride is now recovered from
industrial smokestacks along with other impurities, such as lead,
arsenic, and radioactive compounds.[24]
     This recovered fluoride is known as silicofluoride and is the
type of fluoride added to over 91 percent of fluoridated water. It is
not naturally occurring, as some proponents of fluoridation would
lead us to believe; it is actually classified as hazardous waste.[25]
This hazardous waste would have been costly to dispose of, so an
ingenious marketing campaign convinced the public of the benefits
of fluoridated drinking water. This paved the way for industry to
sell its waste to water utilities.
     To date, all safety studies on fluoride have been conducted
using pharmaceutical-grade fluoride, not industrial-grade
silicofluorides, which have never undergone long-term studies that

116

ensure safety.[26] Perhaps this explains why US EPA scientists are among the most outspoken critics of fluoridation. Approximately 1500 scientists, lawyers, engineers and other US EPA professionals are members of the National Treasury Employees Union, which opposes fluoridation of drinking water supplies.[27]

Sodium fluoride is another form of fluoride, which was the predominant means of fluoridation before the silicofluorides gained the majority of the market share. Sodium fluoride is also commonly found in rat poison and roach control products.[28]

Is There a Better Way to Prevent Cavities?

Cavities are not caused by fluoride deficiency, but can be caused by calcium deficiency, particularly in children exposed to fluoride in their drinking water. Adequate dietary calcium intake is effective at preventing both dental cavities and dental fluorosis. One scientist purports that limiting fluoride in the drinking water to less than 0.5 ppm along with ensuring calcium intake of at least one gram daily is the most effective strategy for the prevention and control of cavities.[29]

Another study showed that for each 5 g of sugar ingested daily, the risk of cavities increased by 1 percent.[30]

A better approach to improving the rate of tooth decay is to cease fluoridation, insure adequate calcium intake in children, and reduce their consumption of sugar and other simple carbohydrates.

What About Fluoride Supplements?

The addition of fluoride to the US water supply has resulted in fluoride accumulation in food products, particularly juice, other beverages, and processed foods. The dose of fluoride obtained from food alone often exceeds recommended levels. This may explain why fluoride supplement use by young children is associated with a substantial risk of dental fluorosis,[31] an indicator of fluoride toxicity.

According to the US CDC, fluoride is only beneficial when applied topically to teeth after they have erupted into the mouth. In fact, the US FDA has never approved fluoride supplements for preventing tooth decay. There is no justification for ingesting toxic fluoride in any form.

Is Fluoride Toothpaste Safe?

Once the permanent teeth have erupted into the mouth, topical fluoride may be beneficial in preventing tooth decay, but independent, unbiased research is needed to validate such claims. Parents would benefit from having definitive answers regarding the benefits of fluoride toothpaste given that there are definite detriments.

Every year thousands of reports of excessive ingestion of fluoride toothpaste, mouth rinses, and other products flood US Poison Control centers. More than 80 percent of children treated for toxic effects of topical fluoride ingestion are under the age of six, the age at which children develop their swallowing reflex.[32] By swallowing even one percent of a tube of children's toothpaste, a child may immediately develop toxic symptoms such as stomach pain, nausea, vomiting, or headaches. Such symptoms often go unnoticed or are never associated with toothpaste enabling continued toxic exposures to occur.[33]

Scientists from the pharmaceutical company, Sepracor, have discovered that fluoridated toothpaste may cause or contribute to loss of teeth. There have also been concerns raised that fluoride toothpaste may cause or contribute to oral cancer.[34]

The US FDA now requires warning labels stating, "Keep out of the reach of children under six years of age" on all fluoride toothpastes and dental care products. Parents are advised to carefully supervise children to encourage spitting and limit toothpaste to a pea-sized amount in order to prevent their children from "overdosing" on fluoride.

Fortunately, there are non-fluoridated alternatives to toothpaste as well as xylitol, which is a natural sugar found to be very effective in preventing tooth decay. It may even help re-mineralize teeth. It is commonly used in Scandinavia for dental hygiene as a topical paste or mint.

Other Sources of Fluoride

To reduce consumption of this toxin, the following lesser-known sources of fluoride may need to be limited as well:[35]

☐ Juice made from concentrate because fluoridated water is often used to reconstitute it. Also true for soda and other processed beverages.

☐ Non-organic grape juice and wine because US grapes are sprayed with a fluoride pesticide called c*ryolite*.

☐ Green and black tea because fluoride from the soil and water is accumulated in the tea plant.

☐ Chicken that is mechanically-deboned to make nuggets often contain ground bone fragments, which contain fluoride.

☐ Salt from countries that fluoridate it.

☐ Some prescription medications contain fluorine. Ask your pharmacist whether your medications do.

☐ Teflon-coated pans may increase the fluoride content of food.

If you are experiencing arthritic complaints, consider eliminating the products above from your diet for one week and see if your symptoms improve. After eliminating green tea from my diet, I had a dramatic improvement in the stiffness of my hands.

Why Water Fluoridation is a Social Injustice

Low-income families cannot afford to buy expensive water filtration devices or bottled water; they are at the mercy of the tap. It is simply not possible for such families to provide fluoride-free water to their children.

Nutrient deficiencies, which increase a child's susceptibility to a host of illnesses as well as to fluoride's toxic effects, are also more likely in low-income communities.[36]

Recent Developments Regarding Fluoride

Some of the more recent statements from the US EPA, FDA, and ADA, which offer hope that the public might regain their right to "choose or refuse" fluoridation are listed below:

☐ June, 2000: A senior scientist at the EPA, Dr. Hirzy, testified about the dangers of water fluoridation before the US Senate; he requested a "moratorium on fluoridation" citing that fluoride is slightly less toxic than arsenic and more toxic than lead.

☐ October, 2006: the US FDA stated that fluoridated water marketed to infants cannot claim to reduce the risk of cavities.

☐ November, 2006: the ADA advised that parents should avoid giving babies fluoridated water because they are at high risk of developing fluorosis.

Despite these recommendations and the enormous body of research regarding its negative effects, the US Department of Health and Human Services, as part of its "Healthy People 2010"" campaign, set a goal of increasing the proportion of the American population served by community water systems with "optimally" fluoridated water by the year 2010.

In an August 2007 statement signed by over 600 professionals released by the Fluoride Action Network, a moratorium to fluoridation was called for. Legislators in fluoridating countries were urged to discover why aggressive promotion to fluoridate continues despite the release of the

National Research Council report in 2006 documenting that its risks clearly outweigh potential benefits. This achievement is felt to mark the beginning of the end of fluoridation around the world.

What Can You Do in the Meantime?

The first step to protect your family from the danger of fluoridation is to determine how much fluoride your water contains. If you have tap water, call the utility and request a copy of the latest water quality report. While you are on the phone, ask if they are adding fluoride to your water or have future plans to do so. If you have well water, you will need to have the water tested yourself.

If fluoride is present in your water, 90 percent can be removed by reverse-osmosis or activated alumina filters. Water distillation also removes fluoride. A carbon filter, such as Brita, will not remove fluoride. It is extremely important to avoid making infant formula with tap water, which delivers a very high dose of fluoride.

Most spring water has less fluoride than tap water. Call the company of the brand you consume frequently to inquire about the source of the water and how much fluoride is in it. Less than 0.1 ppm fluoride is ideal.[37]

Consider non-fluoridated toothpaste for children, particularly if they are under the age of six. Health food stores carry natural alternatives. Your child will love "Silly Strawberry" by Tom's of Maine. If cost is a factor, consider simply using a paste of baking soda.

Consider educating your neighbors and forming a community coalition to petition for the termination of water fluoridation. Remember that some of your neighbors may not be able to afford fluoridation removal or an alternate water supply and your efforts to cease fluoridation may be their only hope to avoid fluoride-related toxicities.[38]

Chapter 15

*H*ome Hazards

"Except in the case of foods, drugs, or pesticides, companies are under no legal or regulatory obligation to concern themselves with how their products might harm human health."
-Alexandra Rome, Former Co-director of the Sustainable Futures Group at Commonweal

Outdoor Environment
It is important to assess whether the environment where you and your loved ones live, work, learn, and play have health concerns. For instance, is your home, work, or child's school located near a polluted lake or stream, industrial plant, freeway, commercial business, dumpsite, or a crop or lawn that utilizes pesticides?

If you suspect a company of polluting your neighborhood, simply go to **www.scorecard.org** and enter your zip code to find out who the biggest polluters are, what they are releasing into the air and water, and what health effects the pollutants may cause. If you don't know who may be polluting your town, you will soon find out! Use this information to mobilize community members to seek protective measures.

If you live in an area with poor air quality it is important to restrict exercise when air quality advisories are in effect. Discuss alternate practice plans with your children's coaches in advance of such days. Try your best to limit the amount of time spent in high traffic areas because diesel fuel and traffic emissions cause more harm than urban smog. Air conditioners and/or air purifiers may help to reduce the negative effect of outdoor air pollution that has penetrated indoors.

If you believe there is an air quality issue in your community, but need proof, consider forming a bucket brigade. Check out **www.bucketbrigade.net** to learn how to collect your own air quality data. Dozens of other communities have used this method to improve pollution and increase enforcement of environmental regulations.

Holler for Your Health

If there is concern about pesticides being sprayed nearby, request notification prior to spraying so you can remove children from nearby playgrounds or other areas that may be affected by pesticide drift. Wineries are notoriously toxic and are a concern if they are located within three miles of a school, daycare, playground, or ball field. Consider persuading such neighbors to switch to organic methods.

According to the WHO, more than 41,000 American deaths annually are attributed to poor outdoor air quality from just one parameter: particulate matter.[1] Yet indoor air quality is a greater concern to health.

When I read that indoor air quality was worse than outdoor air quality I felt certain that this was misinformation generated to deflect concern away from toxic industrial releases. However, after performing additional research I realized that the toxins inside our homes, places of employment, schools, and daycares are, indeed, a significant health threat. This is troubling because of the enormous amount of time we spend indoors, which averages 90 percent, according to the National Safety Council. Fortunately, by making a few changes in our purchasing decisions and daily habits, we can clean up our indoor air, decrease our exposure to toxic products, and eliminate or reduce many adverse health effects.

Take Home Toxins

Many toxins are carried into our homes from the outdoors. While waiting inside a pizzeria for my take-out order, I was enjoying the breeze from the open front door. After a few minutes of fresh air I began to notice a noxious, disturbing odor. I looked toward the door and saw the tailpipe of a vehicle emitting its fumes directly into the pizzeria. I was stunned by the profound difference that idling this vehicle in front of the store had upon the quality of air that I, and all of the other patrons and employees, were forced to breathe.

While searching for a corner of the room with fresher air, I remembered a professor I once had in college. She passionately informed our class about the negative environmental impact of an idling vehicle and admitted that she would reach into such vehicles and turn them off. My classmates and I felt that this action was over the top and joked that she would be arrested one day. As I began to experience the subtle brain fog, irritability, and headache associated with the foul air being pumped into the pizzeria by the uninformed gentleman awaiting his pizza, I finally understood what drove my former professor to take such dramatic action.

How many times have we left the engine running at the drive thru or while waiting for someone or something? These small actions take an enormous toll on the environment and the health of those around us. One simple, yet profound, change we can all make today is to simply turn off our vehicles when running errands or waiting. Avoiding the drive thru whenever possible has the added bonus of burning a few extra calories as you run inside. You will also develop relationships with the employees you meet inside, which can go a long way if you ever need a special favor from your local bank!

Toxins can also be tracked into the home by family members. "Take-home exposures" occur when family members become ill because of the toxins that are carried on the shoes, clothing, hands, or car interiors of workers. Examples of this include lead poisoning among the children of battery workers and cancer resulting from asbestos exposure among families of shipyard workers.[2]

Toxins may also be derived from the soil right outside the door. Arsenic and other toxic wood preservatives, lead from peeling paint, pesticides, weed killers, and other toxic lawn chemicals are commonly found in the soil of most homes, which end up in house dust. A simple solution is to have everyone who enters the home remove their shoes at the door. According to Leo Galland, M.D., the level of toxins in house dust is significantly lower in homes where shoes are routinely removed upon entering. If possible, choose bare flooring in lieu of carpeting, which can trap up to a hundred times the amount of dust.

Toxins can also be carried into the home on dirty hands. And little hands often end up in little mouths. Arsenic from treated wood can be found on playground equipment, decks, and picnic tables. Pesticide residue and lead from playing in the yard may all be present on children's hands. Washing hands is an excellent way to remove these toxins, especially before eating. But, avoid the use of antimicrobial products, which are decimating ecosystems and causing a rise in pathogens that are resistant to antibiotics.

While some toxins migrate into our homes from the great outdoors, others originate from within.

Hidden Hazards in Home Construction

Some dwellings have inherent health concerns due to lead, asbestos, radon, or formaldehyde. For instance, lead was often used in paint prior to being banned in 1978; therefore, children who spend time in older homes may be at risk of lead exposure.[3]

123

The elimination of lead or asbestos from the home, school, work, or daycare should be performed by a professional, and children and pregnant women should avoid exposure to the renovation. Newer studies indicate that there is no safe level of lead exposure. In fact, intelligence drops most strikingly at the lowest levels of exposure with less loss of IQ as lead exposure escalates.[4] Lead has also been associated with aggression and may lead to violent behavior.[5]

Basement or lower level living spaces may contain asbestos or radon, which are both associated with increased lung cancer. Seventeen million US homes are believed to contain unacceptable levels of radon, which is a radioactive gas that may enter the house from the soil. Because radon is more prevalent in certain geographic regions, simply contact your local health department to determine if radon is a factor in your community.[6]

The state of California calls formaldehyde a toxic air contaminant with no safe level of exposure (Proposition 65). Yet it is ubiquitous in indoor environments so reducing exposure is difficult. Formaldehyde is a common component of furniture, cabinets, and other pressed wood or particleboard products. It is also present in carpet adhesive, durable press drapes and permanent press clothing.[7]

Those who spend time in mobile homes are especially vulnerable to this toxic gas because such homes are composed of a plethora of these materials. Many of the children who became homeless after Hurricane Katrina are now complaining of asthma attacks, rashes, fatigue, and severe allergic reactions believed to be a result of living in temporary housing laden with formaldehyde.[8]

Increasing ventilation in rooms with formaldehyde-emitting products is helpful, particularly in the first year of use, since formaldehyde emissions decrease over time. Stiff fabrics, as in new clothing, carpeting and upholstered furniture out-gas for days or weeks while wrinkle-proof clothing will out-gas forever. For this reason, never dress children in wrinkle-proof clothing, wash all clothing before wearing, and air out rooms with new carpeting or upholstery for about a week before allowing children to occupy them. Keeping humidity below 50 percent will limit the disintegration and out-gassing of formaldehyde adhesives. (This will also reduce biological contamination and mold.)

In April 2007, the state of California passed stricter standards regarding formaldehyde emissions for all products manufactured after January 1, 2009. These standards are similar to standards already protecting residents in Japan and the majority of the European Union. Call your legislators to demand similar protective measures in your state. These standards will allow promising nontoxic alternatives such as PureBond, a soy-based adhesive, which is similar in price, to successfully compete in the marketplace.[9]

Indoor Air

Breathing air that is contaminated with tobacco smoke exposes us to nearly 5,000 toxins including benzene. Benzene exposure increases the risk of developing leukemia, which is the leading cause of childhood cancer in the US. In addition to increasing the risk of cancer, tobacco smoke inhalation causes frequent colds, allergies, asthma, and recurrent ear infections. Smoking and environmental tobacco smoke worsens breathing and middle ear symptoms. It also increases the incidence of sudden infant death syndrome, asthma, and lung cancer.[10]

Some states have caught on to the serious health effects of environmental tobacco smoke and have prohibited smoking in restaurants, bars, and other public places. If this is not yet the case in your state, notify your legislator that this issue is important to you. Be sure to declare your home and vehicles smoke-free and ask your workplace or establishments you frequent to move smokers away from doorways. If you are a smoker, give quitting another try. It may take many attempts to succeed, so try, try again.

The heating source of a home is also an important source of potential indoor air pollution. Stoves, heaters, fireplaces, and dryers may emit byproducts of combustion, such as carbon monoxide, wood smoke, and nitrogen dioxide. Carbon monoxide may cause fatigue, headaches, dizziness, weakness, confusion, or nausea at low concentrations and may be fatal at higher concentrations. A carbon monoxide detector will inform you if it becomes a threat. Wood smoke and nitrogen dioxide, which is emitted from kerosene heaters and natural gas appliances, may cause or worsen respiratory illness. Nitrogen dioxide has also been shown to worsen cancer in animals. Emissions can be dramatically reduced by electrical ignition of gas stoves rather than a pilot light. Minimize exposure to combustion products by periodic maintenance of furnaces and by directly ventilating them to the outdoors.[11]

Volatile organic compounds (VOCs) can out-gas into the air where they mingle with dust particles and are often inhaled. Many household products, such as aerosol sprays, household cleaners, disinfectants, stored fuels, automotive products, dry-cleaned clothing, caulk, adhesives, latex paint, polyurethane varnish, vinyl floors, floor wax, furniture polish, moth balls, air fresheners, toilet bowl deodorizers, and plastics emit toxic VOCs into the air. Toxic VOCs are also emitted from computers, printers, and fax machines. Some VOCs are known carcinogens.

To reduce exposure to indoor air toxins:
- ☐ Use a wet rag or mop to wipe down all horizontal surfaces frequently.
- ☐ Vacuum regularly, preferably with a HEPA filter in place. Wear a dust mask and have children play elsewhere.
- ☐ Keep computer equipment out of bedrooms, preferably in a well-ventilated room. Print all documents at once and leave the room while printing.
- ☐ Consider investing in an air purifier.
- ☐ Immediately dispose of excess paint or toxic chemicals. Your local garbage company can provide information about where to dispose of such toxic household wastes.
- ☐ Use artist's paint, paint thinners, furniture strippers, stained-glass making kits, model-building glues, and other toxic chemicals outdoors whenever possible. Increase ventilation and keep children away if using indoors.
- ☐ Never idle a vehicle inside the garage or operate gasoline powered engines in confined spaces.
- ☐ Use a carbon monoxide detector and smoke detectors.
- ☐ Never use a gas oven or range or kerosene heater to heat the house. Families who are struggling to heat their homes properly should be advised to go to social services or seek help from heating assistance programs to prevent the use of alternative heating sources which may lead to poisoning.
- ☐ The following list contains some plants considered to be efficient in removing indoor air pollutants: bamboo palm, Boston fern, chrysanthemum, dwarf date palm, English ivy, ficus, gerbera daisy, golden pothos, peace lily, philodendron, poinsettia, spider plant. [12]

Cleaning Products

A major portion of the 25 gallons of hazardous chemicals used in the home of the average American are household cleaning products.[13] Ironically, cleaning products are making a mess. More than 32 million pounds of these products reach sewage treatment plants daily, overwhelming the ability to remove the toxic substances before the waste enters water bodies.[14] This means more chemicals in our drinking water and more harm to wildlife and ecosystems. The California Department of Fish and Game discovered that the most toxic substances to aquatic life present in their waterways were household bleach, all-purpose cleaner, laundry detergent, and dish detergent.[15]

As with other chemicals, humans are not immune to their effects. Within 26 seconds of exposure, traces of toxic cleaners can be found in every organ of the body.[16] They have been linked to allergies, birth defects, and psychological problems.[17] One eye-opening study revealed that household cleaning products cause three times the rate of cancer than air pollution.[18]

Another problem with these toxic cleaners is accidental poisoning. Every 30 seconds, a child is accidentally poisoned at home.[19] More than 1.4 million Americans, most under the age of six, were referred to poison control centers in 2001 because of household chemicals.[20]

Thankfully, there are many safe, effective, and affordable cleaning products on the market. The Green Guide offers a list of non-toxic cleaners for a variety of cleaning needs (**www.thegreenguide.com**). Because there are no standards for the terms natural or non-toxic, inspect the label to insure the product has no warnings. Ingredients should include a plant-based detergent, such as coconut oil rather than petrochemicals. Grain alcohol should be present as a solvent in lieu of 2-butoxyethanol. Disinfectants should be plant oils such as rosemary, sage, or eucalyptus. Always avoid anti-bacterial products such as triclosan, which are destroying ecosystems, contributing to antibiotic resistance, and confer no health benefit to users.

According to Seventh Generation, a manufacturer of bio-based cleaning supplies, if every household in the US replaced just one bottle of petroleum-based cleaner with an equivalent bio-based product, we would save 118,700 barrels of oil in one year; that's enough to heat 6,800 homes.

If you prefer to save money and make your own non-toxic cleaning supplies, try a mixture of vinegar and water to clean windows, a paste of baking soda to clean the oven and other kitchen and bathroom surfaces, and borax for laundry stains. Search for an online group or forum that shares cost-saving, environmentally-sound secrets such as these.

Arsenic

Arsenic was once a widely used wood preservative in the US. It may be present in decks, playground equipment, picnic tables, park benches, fences, boat docks, or lining flower beds. Most wood used outdoors was pressure treated with arsenic known as chromated copper arsenate (CCA) prior to February 2002.

Arsenic is a known carcinogen; it has been linked to liver, lung, skin, and bladder cancer. It is also a reproductive and immune system toxin and has been associated with diabetes.[21]

Arsenic leaches from the wood into the soil and water. One study showed that soil beneath a CCA treated deck had arsenic levels 2000 percent higher than soil unexposed to the wood.[22] Touching the wood releases the toxin directly into the hands, and often subsequently into the mouths, of children. If edible crops are planted in beds lined with treated wood, the toxin can contaminate the food by migrating up the roots from the soil or water.

Safer Stuff: When buying commercial mulch, be sure to request "virgin mulch," which won't contain CCA treated wood.

The fumes from burning CCA wood are highly toxic. In fact, one tablespoon of its ash contains a lethal dose of arsenic. Never burn treated lumber.[23] Sanding or sawing CCA treated wood releases arsenic into the surroundings. Always wear a mask, gloves, and protective clothing, ensure adequate ventilation, and be certain there are no children in the vicinity.

Although it may have a greenish tint, testing is the only way to know for sure if wood contains arsenic. To order a home test kit (costs about $23) for arsenic go to: **http://www.healthybuilding.net/arsenic/index.html**. If you discover you have CCA treated wood you can either have it replaced or sealed. Sealing the wood every six months with water-based paint or a polyurethane coating will reduce arsenic exposure.

CCA treated wood can be replaced with a variety of products. Naturally pest-resistant woods, such as redwood and cedar are an option if it is salvaged or certified as sustainably harvested. Check out (**www.certifiedwood.com**) or (**www.forestworld.com**) for suppliers. Composites made from recycled materials are another good choice. Examples include ChoiceDek (**www.choicedek.com**), Trex (**www.trex.com**), and CareFree (**www.carefree-products.com**). Healthier preservatives such as borax, sodium carbonate, potash, linseed oil and beeswax are also safer options.[24]

When exposed to CCA treated wood, try to keep food, beverages, and little mouths from contacting the wood. Use a table cloth for picnic tables or have a picnic on the ground (if it has not been treated with pesticides). Insure that children wash their hands after touching hand rails or playground equipment with CCA treated wood, particularly before eating. Do not store toys under treated decks or allow children to play beneath them. Place a blanket or other covering on decks on which children play.

One relatively cheap and environmentally friendly way to remove arsenic from contaminated soil is to plant a special breed of fern, Pteris genus (edenfern™), which actually cleans the arsenic out of the soil. It is capable of removing 10–15 parts per million of arsenic, which is more than 200 times that of any other plant tested. To order go to **http://www.edenspace.com/edenfern-order.htm**. Because of the need to order a fairly large quantity, consider asking your neighbors if they would like to order with you.[25]

Flame Retardants

In order to meet federally mandated fire safety standards, chemical flame retardants have been added to appliances, upholstery, clothing, mattresses, plastics and other products for years. The need for flame retardants began as we shifted to synthetic products, such as petroleum-based plastics, which easily ignite, rapidly disperse flames, and release chemical toxins when they burn. The benefit of preventing these synthetic materials from catching fire is obvious: fire kills more than 3,000 people annually, 600 of whom are children. What is not clear is whether or not we have done more harm than good. Evidence has been mounting since the 1970s that chemical flame retardants have significant negative effects on health, particularly in developing children.[26]

Bromine-containing flame retardants have been categorized as persistent pollutants and subsequently banned from several countries. They have been identified in household dust, food, air, soil, and water samples in the US, Canada, Northern Europe, Taiwan, and Japan.[27] Environmental monitoring programs have found brominated flame retardants in human breast milk, fish, aquatic birds, and elsewhere in places as remote as the Arctic.[28]

Human exposure is highest in the US and Canada, with levels 10–100 times higher than those reported in Europe and Japan. The European Union began replacing brominated flame retardants with alternatives in the 1990s and is now realizing a reduction in levels in breast milk. The Canadian government listed certain brominated flame retardants as toxic in December 2006 and banned their manufacture in Canada. Whether this will result in lower levels among Canadians remains to be seen since they import rather than manufacture these chemicals. American levels are rising.

The US, the world's largest producer and consumer of these chemicals, has no protective measures in place. Perhaps the Swedish ban on these toxic chemicals in the early 1990s, in comparison to the US failure to act, accounts for the dramatic difference in exposure levels.[29] In the absence of federally mandated protections, several states have implemented protective legislation. California and Maine have banned the manufacture and use of certain types of brominated flame retardants, "penta" and "octa," beginning in 2006. Several other states have followed suit.

Fortunately the only US manufacturer of "penta" and "octa," Great Lakes Chemical Corporation (now Chemtura Corporation), voluntarily ceased the production of these types of brominated flame retardants at the end of 2004.[30] The US EPA subsequently instituted the "Significant New Use Rule", which requires that they be notified prior to the importing or manufacturing of these two types of flame retardants after January 1, 2005.[31] Although a step in the right direction, neither of these actions guarantee protection from exposure as these chemicals have not been banned by the federal government. Historically, a voluntary removal of a toxic chemical by industry only allows a window of opportunity for future production of the toxin without regulation. A recent example of this is the high levels of cancer-causing benzene found in soda and juice in 2006. For over 20 years the US FDA failed to monitor industry's voluntary agreement to limit its use.[32] Moreover, the production of the third type of brominated flame retardant, "deca," remains unaddressed.

Worldwide, "deca" continues to be the brominated flame retardant most widely used.[33] The electronics industry has been one of the largest consumers; they are primarily used in the outer casings of computers, printers and televisions. In a US study by The Computer Take-Back Campaign (CTBC) and Clean Production Action (CPA), "deca" residue was found in the dust swiped from every single computer sampled. "Deca" may be a greater problem than currently recognized. It is accumulating in birds and is present in mother's milk.[34]

Brominated flame retardants have similar chemical properties to PCBs.[35] PCBs, which were once commonly used as insulation in electrical transformers, lubricating oil in pipelines, and mixed with adhesives, paper, inks, paints and dyes, are known hormone disrupters and persistent pollutants. They were banned in the US in 1976.

Some evidence is emerging which suggests that, like PCBs, brominated flame retardants may also be hormone disruptors. Animal studies have also revealed adverse effects on brain development including problems with learning, memory and behavior with exposure before or after birth. Exposure during critical points in development adversely affects reproduction, immune system function, and thyroid hormone levels. The possibility of developing cancer is less clear.

Avoiding exposure to these flame retardants is difficult because the chemicals are already ubiquitous in our environment. Limiting the number of products with these chemicals in the home is ideal, but retailers often don't know which products contain them because they are not listed on product labels.

Perhaps a more feasible solution is to reduce or eliminate the need for chemical flame retardants in the first place. Believe it or not, this is possible. Electronics can be designed with components that generate less heat, and flammable components can be separated from heat generating components with increased spacing or metallic barriers. Returning to fabrics that are inherently flame resistant will also eliminate the need for these chemical additives. Metal, leather and glass do not require flame retardants. Natural fibers such as hemp and wool do not require flame retardants either. Reducing our consumption of inherently flammable plastic products will also reduce our reliance on flame retardants.[36]

When a chemical flame retardant is required, less toxic alternatives can be used. The Danish EPA contends that safer alternatives are already commercially available. The German government has identified three flame retardants (aluminum trihydroxide, ammonium polyphosphates, and red phosphorus) that it claims are less troublesome to the environment.[37]

Some manufacturers have voluntarily switched to safer products. IKEA furniture, Crate and Barrel, and Eddie Bauer are using polyurethane foam that is free of brominated flame retardants. IBM, Intel, Motorola, Panasonic, Phillips, Sony, Apple, and Toshiba are also using alternatives in their computers and/or electronics. If we support companies who choose less toxic products and more companies will follow suit.

Pest Control and Lawn Care

"By their very nature, most pesticides create some risk of harm to humans, animals, or the environment because they are designed to kill or otherwise adversely affect living organisms."

-US EPA

According to the US EPA, 80 percent of a typical person's exposure, and the most common means of childhood exposure, to pesticides occurs *inside* the home. Millions of pounds of pesticides are used residentially in the US annually. In urban areas, 90 percent of households use pesticides while 82 percent of all US households use them. Pesticides are predominantly applied within the home, with a smaller amount used in the yard or garden.[38]

Pesticides are found in bug spray, flea shampoo, rat poison, and moth balls. Some shelving paper, paints, and wallpapers may also contain poisonous insecticides or fungicides. Pesticide and herbicide residues are also frequently tracked in from the yard or garden and wind up in household dust. Once inside, there is less sunshine to decompose the toxins, which means they can persist for long periods of time hidden within stuffed toys, furniture, and carpeting.[39]

Several studies show an association between childhood cancer rates and the use of pesticides in the home and yard. Pesticides and herbicides have been found to be toxic to reproduction, development, and the nervous system.[40] Pesticides are especially harmful to infants and pets that spend time close to the ground where pesticide concentrations are highest.

Despite increasing restrictions governing their use, more than 50 percent of all insect killers used by US households are organophosphates.[41] These agents cause damage to developing nervous systems, even when exposures are too low to reveal obvious signs of toxicity.[42] One of the greatest impacts that organophosphates have on maturing brains is the disruption of serotonin systems, which are responsible for maintaining mood.[43]

Fortunately, most household pesticide exposures are avoidable. Start by ceasing to spray lawns and gardens with insecticides, herbicides, or fungicides. The harmful effects of pesticide drift can be mitigated by raising community awareness and requesting that agricultural applications be avoided in windy conditions. Consider alternative flea control products such as pills or injections. Integrated Pest Management is an alternative to toxic pesticides. Go to **www.ipm.org** for more information. If it is necessary to fumigate, arrange to have the children removed from the dwelling for an extended period.

Do not use insect repellant with DEET (N,N-diethyl-meta-toluamide) on children under the age of two and be sure that it contains no more than 10 percent DEET if used on children under five. In older children, apply to the exposed clothing; applying DEET under outerwear is dangerous as it will enhance absorption. Other methods to avoid attracting pests include avoidance of scented soaps and shampoos and wearing long shirts and pants tucked into socks.

The Governor of California passed the Daycare Pesticide Right to Know Act on 1/1/07 to extend the protection of children from toxic pesticides to private day care facilities. (The Healthy Schools Act of 2000 had already covered public facilities.) The new law will require day care personnel to be educated about safer alternatives to pest control and to notify parents and post signs when pesticides are used. Let California's success encourage you to seek similar protective measures in your state. Share this information with your local daycare, school board, or legislators.

Historical Stuff: Chlordane (termite treatment) exposure has been associated with impairment of the nervous system and psychological problems. A 1994 study showed that exposed adults had impaired balance and reaction time as well as mood disorders, lung problems, joint complaints, and behavioral symptoms. Because the central nervous system is the primary target of these insecticides, humans should have never been exposed to them. Chlordane was applied on or around at least 30 million American homes before it was banned in 1987.[44]

Pools and Spas

> **"...You can make a difference by lobbying local officials and pool managers to replace chlorine in public pools with safer, more modern disinfection methods. ...Other alternatives are available and worth exploring. Chlorine disinfection of water is obsolete."**
>
> **-Andrew Weil, M.D.**

Chlorine is highly flammable, hazardous to ingest, breathe, or even handle, yet it is routinely added to our drinking water, pools, and spas. Chlorine gas is an effective chemical weapon because it attacks anything organic, which means any living thing. When chlorine combines with organic matter it forms organochlorides and dioxin.

Organochlorides are toxic pesticides and dioxin is known as the most toxic, most carcinogenic non-radioactive substance known to mankind. According to the US EPA, dioxin is 300,000 times more potent a carcinogen than DDT. Dioxin has also been linked to birth defects, reproductive disorders and infertility, neurological disorders, diabetes, and immune system dysfunction. In 1994, the US EPA listed chlorine on its top 10 carcinogen watch list.

Chlorine byproducts are inhaled or absorbed when showering, bathing, or swimming in water that has been chlorinated. Just opening a dishwasher or sitting beside a pool causes health problems as well. Many household products contain chlorine in the form of bleached paper products such as coffee filters, which leach dioxin into the coffee, and paper-towels, which allow chlorine absorption through the skin.

The toxic byproducts of chlorine are not readily broken down so they persist in the environment and bioaccumulate in the food chain. The average American now ingests 300–600 times the level of dioxin that has been considered "safe" by the US EPA.

Alternatives to water chlorination exist and should be explored.

Chapter 16

*T*he Problem with Plastic

According to The Berkeley Plastics Task Force, the plastic industry contributes 14 percent of the most toxic industrial releases into the air. Plastics, which are never fully biodegradable, make up a large portion of municipal solid waste. Another problem with plastic is that one of its building blocks is petroleum, a non-renewable resource that contributes to our dependence on oil.[1]

Dioxins are produced when plastics are manufactured and incinerated. In addition to being a hormone disruptor, dioxin also damages the immune system, and may affect reproduction and childhood development. In its 2000 report, the US EPA estimated that the average American's risk of contracting cancer from dioxin exposure may be as high as 1 in 1,000.[2] Because of the profoundly negative impact on the planet from plastic production and disposal, it is wise to avoid plastic whenever possible.

Because of our dependence on plastic, this will be difficult, if not impossible. When plastic products are essential, at least know that all plastic is not the same. For this reason, it is important that we familiarize ourselves with the different types and avoid those believed to be most toxic. Fortunately, a code was developed to aid recycling centers in sorting plastics and can be used by consumers to determine what type of plastic a product is made of. If you find the number within a triangle, you can identify the type of plastic.

Plastics by Number

"With your food use 4, 5, 1, and 2, all the rest aren't good for you."
-From the Institute for Agriculture and Trade Policy's Smart Plastics Guide: Healthier Food Uses of Plastic for Parents and Children

Number 1:	Polyethylene terephthalate (PETE or PET)	Used for many transparent beverage bottles
Number 2:	High density polyethylene (HDPE)	Used for milk and detergent bottles as well as reusable food storage containers
Number 3:	Polyvinyl chloride (PVC)	Used for plastic wrap, detergent, and cooking oil bottles
Number 4:	Low density polyethylene (LDPE)	Used for produce bags and baby bottle liners
Number 5:	Polypropylene (PPE or PP)	Used for yogurt and margarine containers as well as plastic squeeze bottles
Number 6:	Polystyrene (PS)	Used for take-out containers or coffee cups. Commonly known by its Dow chemical trade name Styrofoam
Number 7:	Usually refers to polycarbonate (PC)	Used for baby bottles, reusable water bottles, and five-gallon water jugs

Information source from: Doherty, Kieran. *Decoding Your Container. Organic Style.* Page 42. June 2005.

Number 1: Polyethylene terephthalate (PETE or PET)

PETE is commonly used in water and soda bottles, carpet fiber, chewing gum, coffee stirrers, drinking glasses, heat-sealed plastic packaging, kitchenware, plastic bags, and squeeze bottles.[3] Antimony can leach out of PETE bottles. It is generally regarded to have low toxicity and is considered safe. Some evidence exists that antimony is carcinogenic when inhaled, but not when ingested.

Although limited studies exist regarding its safety,[4] one study revealed that antimony was present in concentrations over 12,000 times higher in patients who died from a type of heart failure that has no known cause and often strikes young people (idiopathic dilated cardiomyopathy) compared with those who did not.[5] This may mean that the common plastic soda and water bottle in use today may not be as innocent as we think.

Number 2 and Number 4: High density polyethylene (HDPE) and low density polyethylene (LDPE)

According to the Healthy Building Network, "no plastic is environmentally benign." However, both low and high density polyethylene are believed to be less hazardous to health and have less environmental impact than other plastics.

Milk jugs, water bottles, shampoo bottles, detergent containers and trash bags are often made from HDPE while shrink wrap, produce and bread bags, and packaging for dairy products such as butter and cream cheese are often made from LDPE. HDPE is the most highly recycled plastic. Neither plastic requires the use of toxic plasticizers.

Number 3: Polyvinyl Chloride (PVC)

"Vinyl turns out to be the most environmentally hazardous consumer product on the market."

-Joe Thornton, PhD, Biologist (From Blue Vinyl Documentary by Judith Helfand)

Vinyl, the poison plastic, is the building block of Polyvinyl chloride (PVC), which has been nicknamed the "Watergate of molecules" because it exposes us to more persistent toxic pollutants than any other product.[6] PVC emits VOCs, which are the largest source of dioxin, which is one of the "Dirty Dozen" most toxic chemicals in use today. It is known to cause cancer and is not easily degraded.[7] PVC products also contain plasticizers, known as phthalates, which are known hormone disruptors.

Dr. P. Brandt-Lauf from Columbia University Environmental Medicine believes every molecule of vinyl chloride poses health risks so any exposure, however small, is unsafe.[8] The International Association of Firefighters claims that exposure to a single PVC fire can cause permanent lung damage and that people die from the PVC fumes long before the flames reach them.[9]

Toxic Hairspray: Vinyl chloride was also used as a propellant in hairspray for many years. It was quietly removed from products when its ability to cause cancer was exposed.when its ability to cause cancer was exposed.

Try to avoid buying PVC, which is often identified by the number 3 in the center of a triangle of arrows. Thankfully, some companies such as IKEA, Nike, and Goodrich are voluntarily phasing out the use of PVCs.

Number 5: Polypropylene (PPE or PP)

Polypropylene is used to make cloudy plastic containers such as Rubbermaid containers, yogurt containers, and straws. Although no plastic product is ideal, this is a safer alternative than most.

Number 6: Polystyrene

Polystyrene (PS foam), more commonly known by the Dow Chemical brand name Styrofoam, is used to make egg cartons, to-go containers, and meat trays. The polystyrene plastic expands into its puffy state by injecting it with pentane gas or one of several chlorofluorocarbons (CFCs), which are known to deplete the ozone layer. According to the US EPA, insulation and foam make up the largest portion of CFC use in the US, followed by air conditioners, industrial cleaning agents, and refrigerators.

Toxic chemicals such as benzene and styrene are also used to make PS foam and are a byproduct of PS foam production. Benzene is the most toxic component of PS foam. It is a known carcinogen and is capable of mutating genetic material. Many experts believe there is no safe level of exposure for carcinogenic agents. Short-term exposure to benzene can cause dizziness, headaches, vomiting, convulsions, irregular heartbeat, coma, and

even death. In prolonged exposures, skin scaling, leukemia, and
death may occur.

Styrene is also capable of mutating genetic material. In
addition, it is toxic to the nervous system. Low levels of exposure to
styrene are known to cause irritation of the eyes, nose, and throat.
Higher levels may cause dizziness, difficulty concentrating, memory
impairment, impaired ability to learn, loss of consciousness, brain
damage, and death. If the exposure is prolonged, decreased
fertility, fetal damage, lung cancer, learning impairment, and
shortened lifespan may result. The US EPA has determined that
styrene leaches into food and beverages from PS foam products. In
human studies, 100 percent of fat cells were found to be
contaminated with styrene and 75 percent of breast milk samples
were contaminated.[10]

PS foam is toxic to the environment as well as our health.
PS foam waste occupies 25–30 percent of US landfill space. It will
take 500 years to dissolve one of the 25 million PS foam cups that
are discarded annually. Incinerating PS foam is no better solution.
Burning releases a multitude of dangerous toxins including
benzene, styrene, and dioxin. Although these vapors can be
controlled, many incinerators do not have the financial resources
to operate with these safety controls in place.[11]

Fortunately, alternatives to toxic plastics exist. Eco-foam is
an environmentally friendly alternative to PS foam that is made
from corn starch. It can be used in electronics, as packaging
material, insulation, and to replace plastic plates, cups, and
utensils. Biodegradable plastic products are increasingly available.
Wild Oats Market is using corn-based containers for bulk food
instead of conventional plastic. Newman's Own is one of a growing
number of companies that uses environmentally friendly
packaging. Eco-friendly insulation has been developed by
Manhattan Institute of Technology. It is made from straw, a
renewable, natural resource. It is non-toxic, biodegradable, and
costs less than PS foam.[12]

While visiting a small, family-owned restaurant in my
husband's hometown, I was distressed to see that they were
serving drinks in PS foam cups. My husband politely asked if he
could have a paper cup instead. I apologized to the waitress/owner
for my husband's request by stating that my poor husband
happens to be married to an environmental health writer. She
smiled as she replied that they had just switched to the PS foam
cups because the salesman reassured her they would save money.
She added that she felt a bit uncomfortable with her decision, but
wasn't fully aware of the environmental effects of PS foam. I wonder

how many establishments would choose PS foam if they factored the health and environmental costs into the savings stressed by the PS foam sales force. Unfortunately, the sales force is not likely to disclose such information. Let your local eateries know that you prefer paper products to PS foam or plastic and tell them why. Knowledge truly is power; pass it on whenever the opportunity arises.

Fortunately, PS foam is an easy item to avoid. It is not a toxic ingredient that is hidden within everyday products; when you are using PS foam products, you know it. Here are some simple suggestions for avoiding PS foam.

☐ Ask restaurant personnel to wrap your leftovers in a piece of waxed paper covered in foil or bring your own container with you.

☐ Carry a Pyrex or Corning glass storage container in your car, purse, or briefcase (they come in all shapes and sizes). When ordering out, ask that the food be placed in your own containers.

☐ Carry a stainless steel travel mug or water bottle to use in place of a disposable cup. If everybody carried their own cup, restaurants would save more money on this expense than by choosing PS foam alternatives.

Number 7: Polycarbonate
Polycarbonate is known to leach bisphenol A (BPA), which is a building block for some plastics, pesticides, fungicides, flame retardants, rubber, and polyvinyl chloride. Bisphenol A-based polycarbonate is used in food containers, baby bottles, five-gallon water jugs, reusable water bottles, and eating utensils. It is also used as a coating in paper cartons that hold liquids and in metal cans to prevent the metal from contacting the food contents. BPA is found in dental sealants, pipes, floorings, adhesives, tools, electrical appliances, enamels and varnishes, and other products.

Unfortunately, the chemical structure of BPA is inherently unstable. It decays over time and leaches into food, water, or other substances that it is in contact with. Leaching of BPA is accelerated by heat, the presence of acidic or basic products within, or repeated washing. Once products containing BPA are disposed of, BPA leaches into the groundwater. Indeed, BPA has been detected in rivers and other waterways. Once present in the environment it is not easily degraded.[13]

There have been conflicting reports regarding the toxicity of BPA. The issue has been complicated by the funding of many studies by the American Plastics Council. For instance, the

140

Harvard Center for Risk Analysis released a report that was designed to review previously published studies to determine whether or not BPA posed a health risk. Their findings, based on examining only 19 of 115 available studies, were satisfactory for the American Plastics Council, which funded the study. When the National Toxicology Program reviewed the results in 2002 they reached a different conclusion. They found that BPA was associated with an increase in tumors of the blood cells, testicles, and mammary glands (breasts). The truth is that 94 of the 115 studies revealed significant adverse effects at low dose exposure to BPA.[14]

Many studies show that BPA disrupts the hormone system by mimicking estrogen. Exposure increases the risk of hormone dependent cancers such as breast, prostate, and testicular cancer. It can also cause abnormalities of brain chemistry and behavior, immune system dysfunction, obesity, diabetes, and hyperactivity.[15]

BPA has recently been shown to be dangerous at even low levels. Low levels at crucial periods of development have been proven to cause lifelong reproductive problems including infertility and early puberty. In fact, one study showed that just a single, low dose of BPA caused hyperactive behavior in a newborn rat.[16]

We know that the level of BPA in half the population is higher than the amount known to cause health problems in animals and that BPA was present in over 95 percent of the people tested by The US CDC.[17] Such widespread exposure has been documented in other countries as well. Human fetuses are already exposed to levels of BPA that are known to cause adverse effects on unborn rodents.[18]

Reducing our dependence on plastic products will surely reduce our exposure to BPA. Although it is difficult to eliminate plastic completely, every alternative purchase helps.

Plastic Products

Plasticizers

Phthalates are plasticizers, which are added to some types of plastic to provide flexibility. About 90 percent of plasticizers are used to make polyvinyl chloride (PVC) into its flexible form. PVC cling wrap is used commercially to wrap cheeses and other foods found at the grocery store.[19] Plasticizers easily leach into food and beverages.

Plasticizers have many other uses. Their ability to insulate makes them useful in electrical cables and capacitors. Their flexibility and ability to form a film are useful in a variety of products such as hairsprays, adhesives, caulks, paints, inks, clothing, toys, pesticides, films, food containers, flooring, raincoats, shower curtains, medical devices, children's toys, breast pumps, and detergents.

They are popular in personal care products such as lotions, skin creams, soaps, shampoos, and nail polish because they provide an oily film that is "moisturizing." Virtually all fragrances and perfumes contain plasticizers, yet they are not required to be listed on labels of cosmetic products or fragrances.[20] Because of the wide variety of products that contain them and the lack of labeling requirements, it is nearly impossible to know whether the products you and your children use contain plasticizers.

It is not surprising to find that virtually all humans have detectable levels of plasticizer byproducts in their blood or urine.[21] Data from the US CDC indicates that humans have plasticizer levels high enough to cause health problems and the highest levels are found in children and woman of reproductive age.[22] It is also not surprising that children have some of the highest levels of plasticizers in their little bodies. They drink milk that is sold in plastic containers out of plastic bottles or sippy cups. They play on vinyl floors, chew on plastic toys, and are bathed in products laden with them. US EPA studies show the cumulative impact of different plasticizers leads to an exponential increase in associated harm.[23] In light of this data, the National Toxicology Program has renewed its concerns about exposure for some children and pregnant women.[24]

The chemical structure of plasticizers makes them hard to degrade. However, they are eliminated rather quickly from the body in contrast to lead, mercury, dioxin, or other toxins.[25] While this is certainly good, it makes it more difficult to establish cause and effect. For instance, testing for plasticizer levels in a mother who has delivered a child with a birth defect will not be helpful because the mother may have already eliminated the toxin from her body.

Plasticizers have many toxic effects including hormone disruption, reproductive problems, and birth defects. In 2000 the US National Institutes of Health (NIH) listed them as reasonably anticipated to be a human carcinogen. California's Proposition 65 lists several plasticizers as reproductive toxins. Because of their ability to cause birth defects, women of childbearing age should avoid exposure. Yet pregnant women aren't routinely advised of the danger of plasticizers and even if they are aware of their danger, plasticizers aren't labeled on products so they don't know which products to avoid. So it comes as no surprise that women of childbearing age, who are most likely to use personal care products, perfume, and cleaning products, had plasticizers levels several times higher than the government's safety level.[26] In fact, researchers at the US CDC found evidence of plasticizers in the urine of every single person they tested and the highest levels were found in women of child-bearing age.[27]

Baby Bottles
A recent study by the Environment California Research and Policy Center revealed that all five baby bottle brands tested (Avent, Dr. Brown's, Evenflo, Gerber and Playtex) leached bisphenol A into the liquid within. The levels were as high as those known to cause toxic effects in animal studies.[28]

San Francisco has banned the use of bisphenol A in products intended for children under three years old, but those residing outside of the Bay City are left without protection. Check out **www.newbornfree.com** for a selection of safer baby bottles. They offer BPA free plastic bottles as well as glass bottles, training cups, and other products. Evenflo makes glass bottles with silicon nipples.

Children's Toys
Children often chew on soft PVC toys, which leach toxic plasticizers into their little mouths. In 1998, after extensive press coverage, several US toy manufacturers such as Brio, Chicco, Evenflo, First Years, Gerber, and Safety 1st voluntarily agreed to remove plasticizers from toys intended for the mouth.

In 2002, the US Consumer Product Safety Commission (CPSC) reviewed the data on plasticizers in chew toys and found the plasticizers were more toxic than previously known. Yet instead of calling for a nationwide ban, they simply lowered the "safe" exposure limit by 20 percent. The CPSC's reason for lowering the limit rather than banning it outright was this: They calculated how much of the plasticizer would be ingested by a child chewing on a PVC toy for a certain amount of time. They then observed children to see how long they spent mouthing PVC toys in a day. They concluded that children spent less than 75 minutes a day mouthing these plastics and that this duration of chewing would expose them to the plasticizer in amounts that were within their new "safety" limit.

They used the data from this silly study to conclude that the plasticizers in PVC toys were safe. This point needs clarification: They did not conclude that plasticizers themselves were safe. Indeed, they have been shown to cause harm. Shouldn't the definition of a safe toy should mean a toy that is safe all the time, regardless of how often it is played with? Why should we allow any exposure to toxic toys by playing with wording?

Calling plasticizers "safe in toys" because of the amount of exposure rather than their inherent safety has failed to protect our children. Children have multiple sources of exposure, which increases their dose to unsafe levels. It has already been documented that children have plasticizer levels high enough to cause health problems.

The European Union has steadfastly supported its original ban on soft PVC teething toys since it was issued in 1999. The Japanese government banned plasticizers in toys that might be mouthed by children under the age of six in 2002. At least 14 countries are phasing out or have already banned toxic plasticizers from children's toys. Once again, the US government lags behind other nations in protecting its children.

With no government regulations and no labeling requirements, consumers can never be certain that the toys their children put in their mouths are safe. California recently passed The Toxic Toys bill, which intends to ban the use of six plasticizers from products intended for children under the age of three.[29] While this is a giant step in the right direction it does not address the fact that young children chew on everything, including plastic spoons and sibling's toys. Dolls, action figures, and other toys designed for older children are more likely to contain harmful chemicals because they are not intended for young children. There is simply no place for harmful chemicals in any children's toys.

To limit your child's exposure to plasticizers in toys try these alternatives:

☐ Instead of plastic, choose wooden toys that are sustainably harvested and decorated with soy based paint.

☐ Place an organic cotton washcloth in the freezer to make an excellent (and cheap) chew toy for teething babies. (Remember to omit the fabric softener and use detergents free of dangerous chemicals. Try environmentally friendly brands such as Seventh Generation or Ecover.)

☐ If you must use plastic, look for the label, "PVC free."

☐ Go to **www.healthytoys.org** to see if your child's toys contain PVC or other hazardous chemicals.

Food Containers and Food Wrap

Avoid storing food or beverages in plastic containers; choose glass or ceramic containers whenever possible. Carry a stainless steel coffee mug with a lid as a water bottle in places where glass bottles are not welcome. Never microwave or reheat food in cans or plastic containers.

Almost all commercial grade plastic cling wrap contains harmful plasticizers; these are used to wrap meats, cheeses, etc in the grocery store. While I recommend avoiding deli meat because of its nitrate content, it may be preferable to purchase cheese at the deli counter where it is wrapped in paper. Because it is nearly impossible to avoid purchasing food that is wrapped in plastic, remove it from its wrapper, cut off a thin layer that was in contact with the plastic and then store it in glass, waxed paper, or less toxic plastic.

The Bottom Line

Number 2, 4, and 5 plastic have not been linked to hormone disruption or cancer and are, therefore, the best choices if you must use plastic. Of these safer plastics, number 2 is the most widely recyclable and, therefore, the best for the planet. Keep in mind that the manufacture and disposal of all plastics, including these, is inherently toxic and undesirable.[30]

Whenever possible seek non-plastic alternatives, such as glassware, stainless steel, or earthenware. If you cannot avoid the use of plastic, consider buying recycled plastic products or shopping at resale shops or yard sales so as not to contribute to more plastic production.

Fortunately, a new line of bio-based plastics are now emerging. These "plastics" are actually made out of crops, such as corn or potatoes and are biodegradable. They are known as PLA or polylactic acid. Earthshell and Natureworks are two companies who have begun manufacturing these safer plastics. Consumer demand will assist in replacing more toxic products with these.[31]

I know that eliminating plastic from your daily routine is an enormous task and may not be feasible for everyone. Simply do your best to select less harmful products. If we all do the same, we can dramatically reduce its production.

Chapter 17

Personal Care Products

Cosmetic producers are not required to conduct safety tests and, contrary to popular belief, the US government does not systematically review the safety of personal care products. (This responsibility has somehow been delegated to the Cosmetic Ingredient Review (CIR), which is funded and run by the cosmetic industry's trade association.) Consequently, 80 percent of the personal products in regular use may be contaminated with impurities linked to cancer and other health problems. And because these contaminants are in petroleum-based products they are easily absorbed through the skin where they circulate throughout our bodies.[1]

An online survey in 2004 revealed that every day one in five US adults use products likely to contain all of the top seven carcinogenic impurities commonly found in personal care products. Because they are impurities and not ingredients, these cancer causing chemicals will not be listed in the ingredients.[2]

One of these impurities, 1, 4-Dioxane has been targeted by the US Centers for Disease Control Agency for Toxic Substances and Disease Registry, which recommends it be avoided. The US EPA considers 1, 4-Dioxane a probable human carcinogen and California has placed it on its "Proposition 65" list of chemicals known or suspected of causing cancer or birth defects. This contaminant has been found in numerous personal care products including name brand baby shampoo and baby wash.[3] The Environmental Working Group (EWG) found that 97 percent of hair relaxers, 57 percent of baby soaps, and 22 percent of all personal care products in their Skin Deep database may be contaminated. In the absence of government or industry safeguards, look for the following ingredients that may contain the contaminant: "PEG," "polyethylene," "polyethylene glycol," "polyoxyethylene," "-eth-" (such as sodium laureth sulfate), "oxynol" "ceteareth," or "oleth."[4]

In addition to impurities, the ingredients themselves may not be safe. In 1988, the National Institute of Occupational Safety and Health found that nearly one-third of the chemicals used as cosmetic ingredients have been reported to the US government as toxic substances.[5] In 1997, after discovering ingredients in cosmetics that are suspected of causing cancer, neurological disorders, and birth defects, the US General Accounting Office testified in a US Senate hearing that "cosmetics are being marketed in the United States which may pose a serious hazard to the public." Aside from the presence of known toxins, 99.6 percent of the personal care products analyzed by the EWG contained at least one ingredient that has never even been assessed for safety.[6]

A 2002 study pulled 72 name-brand beauty products right off US store shelves and tested them for a group of toxic plasticizers known as phthalates. Despite the fact that the labels did not reveal their presence, nearly three quarters of the products tested contained these plasticizers.[7] Similar results were found in Europe.[8]

Parabens

Parabens are antimicrobial preservatives that are found in cosmetics, skin cream, sunscreen, shampoo, and even pet food. Parabens may be listed as ethylparaben, methylparaben, propylparaben, benzylparaben, or butylparaben or many other names on labels. A 2004 study identified that all 20 breast cancer samples tested contained paraben. The form of paraben found in the tumors was consistent with a topical route of entry, suggesting that the use of lotions, deodorants, and other personal care products containing paraben are absorbed by and accumulate within the body.[9]

While these preliminary findings suggest that paraben may be a factor in the alarming increase in breast cancer rates, further studies are needed. While further data is being gathered, you will need to decide for yourself whether you wish to be exposed to this known hormone disruptor. If not, you will have to read labels very carefully or go to **www.cosmeticsdatabase.com** and type in the brand of personal care products you use to see if they contain paraben.

Estrogen

Some cosmetics contain the female hormone estrogen. The US FDA does not regulate cosmetics containing less than what is equivalent to an adult dose of hormone replacement therapy (HRT), which has many adverse reactions.

Women taking HRT are often unaware that their cosmetics also contain estrogen, so they may be inadvertently exposed to cumulative doses that increase their risk of side effects.

At the other end of the age spectrum, young girls and

children often use these cosmetics. It is unknown whether these products can cause early puberty, which is very common in African American girls who are significant users of such products.[10] Early puberty is a known risk factor for breast cancer.[11] Interestingly, African girls residing in their homeland, who do not use such products, do not reach puberty prematurely.

Fragrances

Shampoos, soaps, body washes, deodorants, lotions, hairspray, laundry detergents, fabric softeners, and numerous other products that are used on a daily basis contain added fragrance. The word fragrance listed on the label of these products may seem innocent, but 80–90 percent of the ingredients of fragrances are actually petrochemicals and industrial byproducts. Because fragrance formulas are considered "trade secrets," manufacturers are not required to list these noxious ingredients; they simply list "fragrance" instead.

The starter compounds for many fragrances consist of far less innocent sounding ingredients like: turpentine oil, petrochemicals, benzene, phenol, toluene, xylenes, cresols, naphthalene, and cyclopentene.[12] The fragrance added to these starter compounds include a list of ominous sounding chemicals including phthalate plasticizers, the hormone disruptor described in the previous chapter. While some of the ingredients are known toxins, 80 percent have never been tested for human safety.

Fragrances don't discriminate. Their effects are equally harmful to those who are exposed by "second hand smelling." When you apply perfume, plug in an air freshener, burn a scented candle, or spray an air freshener, you are exposing everyone who is forced to breathe the air, to the chemicals it contains.

The Institute of Medicine classifies fragrance and second hand smoke in the same category for ability to trigger asthma. This is no small matter considering that 26.3 million US citizens are afflicted with asthma. In many cities, potentially deadly asthma attacks are the leading cause of emergency room visits for children.

Fragrances have also been linked to skin rashes, kidney damage, liver damage, immune system dysfunction, chronic illness, stomach complaints, blood pressure changes, and brain and nervous system disorders such as headaches, depression, dizziness, memory loss, impaired concentration, panic attacks, anxiety, insomnia, impaired vision, spaciness, giddiness, slurred speech, and loss of muscular coordination.[13] Studies on mice revealed an impact on the respiratory and nervous systems when exposed to fragrances in everyday products, such as air fresheners and fabric softeners.[14]

About 20 percent of Americans have adverse reactions to the scent of perfume or other fragrances. Infants, children, pregnant women or women of reproductive potential, the elderly, those with weakened immune systems, and those who are sensitive to chemicals are most likely to be negatively affected by fragrance. Such considerations once prompted the state of California to propose a bill banning perfume in the workplace.

As in all things we do, we should consider the impact on our neighbors. We certainly wouldn't consider spraying a toxin in the face of a child then sending him to the ER with a potentially deadly asthma attack; we wouldn't willfully expose a mother battling breast cancer with a substance that would weaken her immune system; and we wouldn't knowingly expose a pregnant woman to a substance that could result in birth defects.

Please think twice before applying that not-so-innocent dab of perfume. Essential oils are a safe alternative to fragrances; many health stores carry these scents.

What is Being Done?

In September 2004, the European Union began prohibiting the use of known or suspected carcinogens, mutagens, genetic mutators and reproductive toxins from cosmetics. US Consumer watchdogs demanded protection as well. In 2005 the US FDA responded to these demands not by banning toxins, but by warning the cosmetic industry to inform consumers that personal care products have not been safety tested. Once again, the US staunchly protects corporate pocketbooks while lagging behind other nations in protecting its citizens from toxins.

In the absence of federal protective measures, some states are picking up the slack. California is once again the forerunner in legislation to protect its citizens from toxic exposures. Despite tough opposition from large cosmetic companies, California passed legislation in October 2006 requiring cosmetic companies to notify the state when they use ingredients linked to cancer and birth defects.

Additionally, 500 companies have heeded the public outcry and have pledged to remove dangerous chemicals from their products by signing the "Compact for Safe Cosmetics." Most of the brands found in drug stores, supermarkets and beauty stores have not signed the pledge. Instead of making their products safer, they have chosen to join the Cosmetics Toiletry and Fragrance Association in an effort to combat protective legislation and

149

unleash a marketing campaign portraying their toxic products as safe.

What Can You Do?

The Environmental Working Group's Skin Deep Database is a terrific website that enables a search for healthier products. Go to **www.cosmeticsdatabase.com** and search for the products you use to see if they contain toxic ingredients. Or use an advanced search; check all of the boxes to exclude products with health and environmental problems and see a list of products that are healthier alternatives for both you and the planet. Nearly 30 million searches have already been performed on this site. This is very encouraging. Each time a consumer selects a healthy alternative over a toxic one, a message is sent to the corporate world saying that we will only pay for safe products. It is time to speak their language. Log on to the Skin Deep Database and find a new brand of shampoo, lotion, and sunscreen.

Chapter 18

*T*echnology

Radiation is energy generated by particles in motion. This motion may be simple vibrations or wave-like oscillations. The electromagnetic spectrum classifies types of radiation by its energy level: the faster the oscillation, the greater the energy. The electromagnetic spectrum is divided into energy that is sufficient to bump electrons off atoms (ionizing radiation) and energy that is not sufficient (non-ionizing radiation).

Ionizing Radiation

Radioactivity, nuclear processes, and x-rays are known sources of ionizing radiation that damage any molecule or atom in its path. But any form of radiation can be ionizing (capable of damaging cells), if it has high enough energy. An example of this is the sun—a form of ultraviolet radiation. The extreme heat generated by the sun imparts sufficient energy to bump off electrons in skin cells of a person who is exposed to its rays.[1] The initial damage this causes is sunburn; the long-term effects may include wrinkling, premature aging, and cancer.

By bumping electrons, ionizing radiation creates unstable charged particles called free radicals that aggressively seek to bond with oppositely charged particles to regain a stable neutral charge. These free radicals are known to wreak havoc on the human body leading to a host of illnesses including heart disease, strokes, and cancer. The energy imparted to human cells by ionizing radiation is capable of destroying our genetic material and the genetic mutations caused by this process can be passed on to subsequent generations. Fortunately, the human body was designed to heal itself and can correct mutations to the DNA or induce the mutated cell to die so its altered DNA cannot be passed on. For this reason, the risk of hereditary diseases or birth defects is considered to be very low.[2] However, long-term or excessive exposures may overwhelm the body's natural protective abilities.

Lead, concrete, or water are suffcient barriers to ionizing radiation. Shielding yourself with one of these barriers will greatly reduce exposure. This is why doctors and nurses wear lead shields when performing procedures that utilize radiation and why a lead shield is placed over your reproductive organs during X-rays.

Excluding unavoidable background radiation sources, by far the greatest exposure to ionizing radiation results from medical procedures. The following recommendations will help lower your exposure:

☐ Avoid whole body scans, which expose the body to almost 100 times the level of radiation of a mammogram.

☐ Limit the use of x-rays, CT (CAT) scans, and fluoroscopy (i.e. cardiac catheterization) unless absolutely necessary. Consider MRI instead of CT scans if possible.

☐ Delay screening mammograms until after menopause, but only if your doctor agrees that the risks outweigh potential benefits of early mammography.

A report released by the National Research Council (the BEIR VII report) in 2005 indicated that background sources of radiation, which are considered unavoidable in modern life (i.e. cosmic rays and nuclear power plants), were associated with a relatively low overall cancer risk.

Non-Ionizing Radiation

Although non-ionizing radiation is not strong enough to dislodge electrons, it is sufficient to cause vibration, excitation, and heat. Examples include radiofrequency microwaves such as mobile phones, TV transmitters, radar, satellite, and other forms of telecommunication and extremely low frequency waves such as power lines, electrical wiring, and home appliances.

Mobile Phones, Baby Monitors, and Cordless Phones

When I was in college, we didn't have cell phones. We didn't even have phone lines in our dorm rooms; we had hall phones. Phone calls were answered by anyone who happened to be passing by a ringing phone and was kind enough to retrieve the recipient. Rather than calling, friends would stop by each other's rooms and leave a message on their door. The convenience of having access to everyone at the push of a button is very new.

Try telling this to a teenager. I remember how foreign it sounded to me when my parents explained that "back in the day" people didn't have home phones (or TV). In the absence of home phones, rare emergency calls were directed to a neighborhood store and a messenger was dispatched to relay the news. The times have most certainly changed.

Technology

There are now nearly 3 billion users of mobile technology worldwide. Mobile phones have become an ordinary part of life. When something becomes as commonplace as a mobile phone, it is hard for a generation who never knew life existed without it, to believe they may be dangerous. But the truth is that technology has exploded at such a rapid pace that our ability to ascertain the safety of widely accepted products lags behind.

Mobile phones emit electromagnetic energy. Although we can't see this energy, it is capable of inducing an electric current. Whether this current causes health concerns has been hotly debated. Newer studies are beginning to reveal that earlier perceptions of safety may have been premature. The following are some emerging health concerns attributed to mobile phones:

☐ Genetic Mutations: Cell phones damage DNA and chromosomes, even at exposure levels currently considered safe.[3]

☐ Cancer: The first well designed study to confirm the suspected link between cancer and cell phones was a 1997 study by Dr. Michael Repacholi and his colleagues, which revealed long-term exposure caused an increase in the occurrence of lymphoma in mice. Another study showed that less than 10 years of cell phone use raises your risk of brain cancer by 20 percent, while greater than 10 years increases risk by 80 percent.[4]

☐ Acoustic Neuroma: Six or more years of cell phone use causes a 50 percent increase in acoustic neuroma, a tumor of the nerve that links the ear to the brain. Although considered benign, it can lead to permanent hearing loss and may be life threatening if untreated.[5] A small Swedish study linked its development with 10 years of exposure.[6]

☐ Headache: The longer the exposure, the greater the incidence of headaches. Fortunately, using hands-free equipment reduces their occurrence.[7]

☐ Impaired Brain Blood Flow: The electromagnetic field emitted from mobile phones while in use decreases blood flow in the region of the brain where the phone is held. This may cause damage to brain cells that rely on such blood flow for vital oxygen delivery.[8]

☐ Brain Damage: Teenagers, whose brains are undergoing maturation, are frequent users of mobile phones. A study of rats, whose brains were of similar developmental stage, revealed that radiation from the phones damaged brain cells. The damage increased with increased duration of exposure. The effects of decades of mobile phone use may result in premature degenerative brain diseases.[9]

☐ Heart and Kidney Damage: Oxidative stress induced by mobile phones has been shown to damage both the heart and kidneys.[10]

☐ Impaired Reaction Time, Memory Disturbances, and Sleep Disorders: These have also been reported.

Newer baby monitors that utilize digital technology have been associated with irritability, crying, and disturbed sleep in infants. Replacing such monitors with older analogue versions or eliminating their use altogether resolves the problem.

Digital cordless phones have recently been upgraded to a higher frequency (2.4 GHZ to 5.8 GHz) because home wireless networks have cluttered the lower frequency ranges. These newer bases release continuous magnetic fields even when the phone is not in use or in the cradle. Sleep disturbances and chronic fatigue syndrome have been seen in adults who have digital cordless phone bases/chargers near the bed. Moving the charger away from the bed or preferably to an area of the home where less time is spent, such as a hallway, will often resolve these complaints.[11]

Power Lines and Home Appliances
There has been much debate regarding the health effects of high voltage power lines and other sources of extremely low frequency electromagnetic fields such as TVs, computer monitors (including laptop computers), fluorescent lights, light dimmer controls, hair dryers, and improperly grounded equipment. As with mobile phones, recent studies are confirming health problems that were previously discounted.

A 1996 review of scientific literature by the National Resources Council revealed that children living in homes with a high electromagnetic current are more likely to develop leukemia. Children exposed to magnetic fields greater than 3 mG had 72 percent more cancer than children living in homes with levels less than 0.65 mG.[12] In 2001, the International Agency for Research on Cancer (IARC, a WHO agency), and the National Institutes of Health, both classified extremely low frequency electric and magnetic fields as possibly carcinogenic to humans.[13]

The California Department of Health Services conducted its own review of the scientific literature and concluded that in addition to increased risk of both childhood and adult cancers, there is an increased risk of miscarriages, suicide, Alzheimer's disease, sudden cardiac death, and Lou Gehrig's Disease (amyotrophic lateral sclerosis) associated with exposure to electromagnetic fields from power lines, wiring in buildings, and household appliances.[14]

The best way to prevent health concerns from electromagnetic fields is to maintain a safe distance from sources. Both electric and magnetic fields diminish with increasing distance from the source. Safe distances are as follows:

- Household Appliances: 3–4 feet
- Transformers: maintain a greater distance from these than other appliances
- Distribution Power Line: 60–200 feet (at least half the width of a football field)
- Transmission Power Line: 300–1000ft (1 to 3 lengths of a football field)

What are Transformers? Transformers convert the high voltage electricity from primary distribution lines to the lower voltage carried by secondary distribution lines to consumers. Transformers look like cylinders on utility poles or boxes for underground lines. High voltage transmission lines are distinguished from community distribution lines because they are usually on metal towers. High voltage transmission lines carry electricity from generation plants to local substations, which then transport the electricity to residences and businesses via distribution lines, which are usually on wooden poles.

Unfortunately, about 10 percent of US schools are close enough to high-voltage power lines to increase childhood cancer risk and up to 4 of 100 children worldwide reside in homes that exceed electromagnetic field levels that have caused health concerns.[15] The good news is that electrical fields are easily blocked by trees, shrubs, and buildings. Magnetic fields, on the other hand, penetrate structures; therefore, they are a greater cause for health concerns.[16] If you are concerned about excessive magnetic fields in or around your home, workplace, or child's school or daycare, purchase a gaussmeter for measuring magnetic fields. Levels greater than 3 mG may be harmful. There are many resources on the web for purchasing a gaussmeter. For example, **http://www.lessemf.com/gauss.html** has a $25 model.

Additional suggestions to reduce exposure to electromagnetic radiation include the following:

☐ Keep mobile phones away from your head. A 1998 study showed that holding a mobile phone against your ear doubles the risk of dying from brain cancer than using a car phone with an external antenna.[17] Hands-free options may transmit radiation into the earphone so loudspeakers may be better. Or consider using a 1 cm thick foam spacer between the phone and your ear.

☐ Limit the use of mobile phones. Ask your teen to text rather than speak with friends.

☐ Choose a phone with the lowest radiation level. Ask to see the manual of several phones to compare.

☐ Keep the phone away from your body. Do not place it in your pocket or attach it to your belt.

☐ Use the Low-Power Standby mode rather than screensaver on computer monitors. Screensavers will not reduce radiation or power consumption. To make this change, simply go to Settings>Control Panel > Display Properties > Screen Saver, and then check the Low-Power Standby box or select the time you wish to turn off the monitor automatically. When the keyboard is idle for the number of minutes you select, the monitor powers down and emits almost zero radiation. Simply touching the keypad or mouse reactivates the monitor.

☐ Suggest computer shielding to your employer and/or school board. This is particularly important for computers in rows (as in a classroom setting) because exposure is highest from the rear of the computer screen.

☐ Choose appliances with a higher Energy Efficiency Rating, which generally produce lower electromagnetic fields.

☐ Unplug appliances when not in use. Anything involving electricity will emit both an electric field and a magnetic field. Magnetic fields are only present when an appliance is turned on, but electric fields are present whenever an appliance is plugged in.

☐ Rearrange furniture so that appliances are not located near sitting areas or beds.

☐ Plant trees or shrubberies between power lines and your home.

Chapter 19

*V*accinations

"Autism is a national economic and spiritual emergency, one that will tear the very fabric of society if we let it. It is a world emergency, and we need to start treating it as such."
-Andrew Wakefield, Executive Director of
Thoughtful House

Claire and Kyle

"Please send my son home exhausted!" were the words Claire wrote to her son's teacher on his first day of kindergarten. They were words she often repeated throughout his schooling; words that reflect the enormous effort required of those who care for and love a challenged child; words that reflect her dire need for a few moments of peace. Claire couldn't have possibly imagined, nor can any of us who have not walked a mile in her shoes, the extraordinary ways in which the bond of love she held for her child would be tested each day of their harried and hectic lives.

Kyle entered this world tipping the scales at ten pounds, six ounces of pure atomic energy. His mother instinctively knew that this squirming, demanding infant was going to be different. His urgent cries and demands were foreshadowing for what was to become a lifetime of agonizing tantrums. On the day Kyle crossed the threshold into his loving home, Claire already arrived at the end of her rope. "I can't take it anymore! He never shuts up! He wants to nurse all day! He wants to be rocked all day! He wants to stay awake all day!"

Each day Claire would regroup and tackle the next day's horrors as only a loving parent can. Despite ear splitting screams and desperate pleas with Kyle's pediatrician who refuted Claire's beliefs that her child must be suffering from colic, she carried on. Each day was a new test of her love for her son. Claire recalls, "I can't tell you how many times I have wanted to quit this motherhood duty."

Kyle doesn't have a physical disability that you notice, unless you look closely. A careful observer may notice that he

157

avoids eye contact and has a robotic manner of speaking. Claire is thankful that Kyle doesn't suffer from severe physical challenges. But when strangers look at the two of them with disdain, she sometimes wishes he exhibited more obvious physical abnormalities. People who are unfamiliar with the pair often cast judgmental looks when they see a robust boy screaming furiously and squirming erratically while his desperate, disheveled, and perspiring mother struggles to quiet him. People witnessing such tantrums often believe her to be an incapable mother with a spoiled brat of a child.

Her son is not a brat. He is not spoiled. He suffers from hyperactivity, obsessive-compulsive behavior, rage and defiance, mood swings, self-isolation, and social immaturity. He is a child with Asperger's syndrome, an autism spectrum disorder (ASD) of which the most severe form is autism. His mother describes keeping up with him as trying to "outrun a marathon runner with hundred-pound weights attached to your ankles."

His inquisitive nature, a result of his genius level I.Q., results in nonstop questions from the moment he wakes up until the moment he passes out. Claire's response to how she endures this endless barrage of questions reflects the humor she has learned to rely on for strength, "for some reason my doctor won't prescribe *me* drugs!"

Children with Asperger's syndrome are often ignored or harassed by their peers. When he was young, Kyle and his mother were "politely" asked to leave a playgroup. Claire recalls, "The scornful eyes of those mothers have left burning imprints on my back. I was shunned; left to play with my child alone, to nurture, love and mold him just the same as his siblings."

For all the love Claire bestows upon her son, little affection is returned. Displaying affection is another quality that has been trampled by the Asperger's syndrome. In lieu of outward signs of affection, Claire relies on "warm and funny memories of survived antics" to revitalize her. Despite all the obstacles, Claire is aware of an "unusual love bond" between her and her son.[1]

Many Children Suffer the Same Fate

The plight of Claire and her son Kyle is becoming increasingly common. The first cases of autism were described by psychiatrist Leo Kanner in 1943 among children born around 1931, the same year that vaccinations were introduced in the US.[2] Autism then began its explosive growth: 1 in 5000; 1 in 500; 1 in 166; and now 1 in 150.[3] In California, which began tracking autism before the rest of the nation, the number of people living with full-syndrome autism has increased by 634 percent between 1987 and 2002.[4] California is not alone. All states have had increases of at least 500 percent over similar time spans. Autism has become an epidemic in industrialized nations, led by the United States and the United Kingdom.

There's No Such Thing as a Genetic Epidemic

Autism is an epidemic. There are people who will vehemently deny this, stating the means of reporting or diagnosing has changed in recent times. While the diagnostic criteria may have changed, a new problem with a new cause has clearly emerged placing an unprecedented burden on families, schools, and communities.

Epidemics are not caused by genetic abnormalities, which are passed down through families. Genetic illnesses emerge slowly over the course of generations. Autism has had an explosive onset. Although genetic factors may be present, there must be another factor. This is good, because it means we can prevent autism by identifying and eliminating or modifying this external factor.

Mercury is a well-known brain toxin and is considered one of the most toxic substances in existence. According to the Agency for Toxic Substances and Disease Registry, mercury's harmful effects "... include brain damage, mental retardation, incoordination, blindness, seizures, and inability to speak. Children poisoned by mercury may develop problems of their nervous and digestive systems as well as kidney damage."[5]

Astonishingly, unsafe amounts of mercury have been injected directly into the bloodstream of infants while their parents have stood beside and watched. Would you willfully inject this poison into your child's bloodstream? I wouldn't, but I did.

Blind Faith

My daughter received her first shots in the hospital on the day she was born. I suppose I must have consented to that, but I don't recall. I am pretty sure I would have remembered, and am absolutely sure I would have refused, if I had been warned of a possible link to autism.

During my daughter's one-month well child check I was handed the mandatory pamphlets regarding vaccinations. I had no reason not to trust the federal government or the pediatrician's recommendations. So I merely glanced at them and returned to the near catatonic state common among new mothers struggling with sleep-deprivation, post-partum hormonal flux, and the stress of managing multiple new roles. If I had a suspicion that there may be a problem I certainly would have paid more attention. Even so, I am not sure that reading the pamphlets would have changed my mind. The information doesn't say my child could become autistic. Besides, my trusted pediatrician looked me in the eye and reassured me it was in the best interest of my child.

And so I willfully allowed my child to be injected with a potent brain toxin. How was I supposed to know the vaccinations were preserved in thimerosal, a form of mercury? Even without that knowledge, my gut told me something was wrong. I felt like I was leading a sheep to its slaughter. My daughter was playfully looking me in the eye with a big toothless grin when all of a sudden she was attacked with the piercing sensation of needles. Her face wrinkled up as she shrieked in terror. I had to stifle my sobs. I knew this little baby had never felt pain before. Would she have nightmares now that she knew pain and couldn't possibly anticipate when it would come next? I felt like such a hypocrite. I cooed at her and played along as if everything was fine when all along I knew what was coming next.

Like me, parents are now forced to stand by and watch their smiling, innocent, helpless little babies as they are pierced with four or more needles in one sitting. And the number of mandatory vaccinations continues to grow. Why so many shots? I thought vaccinations were intended to prevent children from crippling diseases like polio or to end deadly epidemics like smallpox.

I was naïve. As the nurse hovered over my screaming child with needles, it never occurred to me that decisions are not always made in the best interest of our children. I had no idea that the vaccination business is a $10 billion dollar industry with lots of influence. I am haunted by my ignorance. I am not just a mother who exposed her child to toxic mercury; I am a mother who exposed countless other people's children to it as well. Just as I had trusted my daughter's pediatrician, these good parents had trusted me.

I remember the first time I heard a campaign against vaccinating children. It was my first year of practice as a physician assistant in a rural family practice setting. I went to a presentation at a local chiropractor's office because I was eager to help people and wanted to know what they could offer my patients. When I arrived, we were shown a video that advised parents of the harm of vaccines. The video encouraged parents to avoid vaccinations. I was outraged; I thought this chiropractor was irresponsible.

But the chiropractor was right. I was wrong. That was 1996, a year in which children were receiving enormous dosages of mercury in their vaccination schedule. I had become a medical provider because I wanted to help people, particularly children. I had been one of the best students in my class. Yet in my naivety I exposed countless children to the potential of unfathomable harm. I am appalled by my own ignorance. I am appalled at the way I, and other medical providers, have been trained. So please don't judge your medical providers and one another; we have all been misled. We are all at different places on the learning curve.

What I Have Learned About Vaccinations

"It is insane to think that injecting a neurotoxin into newborn babies will have a beneficial effect..."
- David Kirby

Vaccinations are not to blame for autism. At least that is what the US CDC has led us to believe. They claim there is no proof that autism is caused by vaccinations. But as a parent who is aware of how difficult it can be to trace a problem back to its cause, I am not interested in whether there is proof of harm; I am interested in whether there is proof of safety.

I know there has been no proof of safety. I also believe there has been proof of harm. Convincing government or corporate officials of the existence of a disease "cluster" and then determining its cause has historically proved futile. However, because autism is now so pervasive, identifying a "noncluster," or a group of children who are not developing autism, may be more fruitful in determining a cause.

Fortunately, nonclusters have been identified. The Amish Mennonnites have only had three children identified with autism in their community. Another noncluster was identified in Cook County, Illinois. What these two nonclusters have in common is that nearly all of the children are unvaccinated. Dr. Mayer Eisenstein, director of Homefirst Health Services, cannot recall a single case of autism among the unvaccinated 30,000 plus Cook County children they serve.[6] Of the three autistic Amish children: one was adopted from China and had received vaccinations in both countries, another became ill immediately after being vaccinated, and the third child's immunization status is unknown.[7]

While this absence of autism in populations that have not been vaccinated may not be deemed sufficient evidence by some, my gut instinct tells me it is. Unvaccinated children are not getting autism in the astonishing numbers that vaccinated children are. The first cases of autism were documented in the first group of children ever to receive mercury in their vaccines. The explosive growth of autism cases correlates with the timing of additional vaccines and therefore increased exposure to mercury, a known brain toxin. What does your gut tell you?

The Science Behind It All

Autism is one of a spectrum of disorders. Likely, there is a spectrum of causes as well. Newer research suggests that autism spectrum disorders are most likely triggered by a chemical or infectious cause in children that are genetically vulnerable to such triggers. The trigger may be cumulative from many sources or may be the result of one profound toxic exposure.[8] This may explain the difference in presentation among children. According to Bryan Jepson, M.D., "Plenty of parents report a gradual deterioration, but many kids seem to develop autism after a particular event. They go into the hospital or they get an MMR (measles, mumps and rubella) shot and they're never the same again."[9]

I was under the impression that children were born with autism and had developmental symptoms from birth. It never occurred to me that the essence of a child could be abruptly stolen from their loving family at two or three years of age. My eyes were opened to this shocking truth when The Oprah Winfrey show aired "The Faces of Autism" in April, 2007. A shocking video of a little boy affectionately hugging his little brother and speaking clearly was followed with a video of the same little boy after receiving mercury-containing vaccinations. The difference was shocking and heartbreaking.

Scientists have now identified a genetic defect involving a substance called glutathione that may predispose certain children to autism and other ailments. Glutathione is required for the body to properly breakdown and eliminate medications and toxic substances. Glutathione is also an important antioxidant. Antioxidants combat oxidation, which may be caused by radiation, medications, pollutants, infection, stress, poor diet, and injury. Oxidative stress further reduces glutathione levels and leads to cellular aging, disease, and death.[10] Glutathione is also important in maintaining proper immune function and protecting the lining of the gut from damage.

According to Dr. Jill James, a former US FDA research scientist who now works at the University of Arkansas for Medical Sciences, autistic children have 133 percent more "inactive" glutathione and 68 percent less "active" glutathione in their bodies than healthy children.[11]

Essentially, autistic children likely have a genetic predisposition for lower levels of glutathione. Therefore, they can't rid their bodies of toxic substances as well as other children. This makes them far more vulnerable to the toxic effects of chemicals. Dr. Mady Hornig of Columbia University discovered that mice with genetically susceptible immune systems displayed autistic-like behaviors when given the same mercury preservative used in vaccinations.[12] Another study revealed that doses of mercury lower than those children received from vaccinations during the 1990s inhibited detoxification processes by over 50 percent.[13]

It appears that genetically susceptible children may develop autism and other developmental disorders as a result of environmental triggers. But why are significantly more boys afflicted with developmental problems, such as autism, than girls? One study showed that nerve cells treated with estrogen had less cell death while nerve cells treated with testosterone had increased death when the mercury preservative was added.[14] The reason for this is that estrogen, found predominantly in females, has been shown to increase glutathione levels conferring greater protection to girls against toxic threats. Estrogen is also an antioxidant like glutathione, providing girls with a larger arsenal to ward off toxins.[15]

Children who were born between 1991 and 2003 received 25 micrograms of mercury in the hepatitis B shot on the day they were born. Many of these children received a total of 187 micrograms of mercury in their first six months of life by following the recommended vaccination schedule. This is well over the level considered safe for adults, but was given to infants whose immune system and detoxification systems weren't fully developed. This excessive toxic exposure may have pushed some of the more vulnerable children over the edge resulting in autism or other developmental problems.[16]

Even if this early toxic exposure does not result in illness, the toxins start to accumulate. As the child is hit with more and more toxins in the form of more vaccinations, medications, and other environmental exposures, his body and sensitive nervous system may become overwhelmed leading to sickness.

A Grave Mistake

Mercury was added to vaccinations as a preservative in 1931. Prior to its standard use in vaccinations, only one "safety" study was performed. It was injected into the bloodstream of 22 patients who were all suffering from terminal meningitis. They all died. The conclusion from the study stated that none of the subjects suffered a life-threatening allergic reaction upon administration. Somehow the researchers used this evidence to deem it was safe. From that point on we began injecting it into our infants and young children.

In 1982 an expert panel at the US FDA reviewed the mercury used in vaccinations and found that it was toxic and caused cell death.[17] Ignoring this data, the US CDC, in 1990, mandated additional shots be added to the current regimen.

I was taught that benefits should outweigh risks whenever medicine intervenes in health. Yet nobody bothered to calculate the risk. Nobody did the math. In *Evidence of Harm,* David Kirby reveals that a pharmaceutical company finally did the math in 1991. But they never bothered to share the horrific results. That is until 1999, when Congress mandated that mercury in medicines be reviewed by the FDA.[18]

The data that was withheld between 1991 and 1999 revealed that infants were administered mercury at levels 125 times the EPA safe exposure level for adults![19] And this was being injected directly into their little bloodstreams.

In 1999, The Agency for Toxic Substances and Disease Registry (ATSDR) advised, "Keep all mercury-containing medicines away from children." Yet, they never bothered to recall the vaccines. The transition to mercury-free vaccinations was not complete until early 2002, and even then our precious children continued to be administered these known brain toxins until the supply ran out. Because shelf life is two and a half years, children may have been exposed through the end of 2004, five years after the ATSDR advised that mercury-containing medications be kept away from children. Incidentally, veterinarians removed mercury from animal vaccines in the early 1990s because of its toxicity.[20]

Why were these toxic vaccines not recalled even after they themselves issued a warning regarding their safety? This resulted in exposing more children to high doses of mercury for several more years. According to Robert F. Kennedy, Jr, "The US CDC failed to make child safety its priority...Will we hold the US CDC accountable for knowingly placing children at risk of neurological injury?"

While the elevated level of mercury once present in vaccines is now undisputed, there is an ongoing debate about whether it has led to the epidemic of autism. Interestingly, neurodevelopmental disorders, such as autism and ADHD, have similar symptoms to those of mercury poisoning and children with autism have been found to have more mercury in their bodies than other children.

Vaccinations

The US CDC hired the Belgian scientist Thomas Verstraeten to study the rate of autism in relation to mercury exposure. His findings were alarming. Children who received more than 25 micrograms at one month of age had 7.62 times the rate of autism as children who received none. A rate of 2.0 or more is considered causation.[21] Because they were responsible for the promotion of the vaccination program, the US CDC was not happy with these findings. The US CDC asked Verstraeten to reorganize his study. By selectively including and excluding certain children, he succeeded in getting the rate increase down to 2.48, but that still implicated mercury as a cause of autism. This prompted additional tampering with the study design until they finally succeeded in getting an autism rate of 1.69. This number allowed the US CDC to report that mercury in vaccinations did not cause autism.[22]

Based on this flawed study, the Institute of Medicine denied the link between vaccines and autism. They went so far as to recommend that the government stop pursuing mercury in vaccines and channel funds and research to other more "promising areas." With so many questions left unanswered, why would they have denounced further research? The bottom line seems to be that the US CDC, which had many conflicts of interest with vaccine manufacturers, made a grave mistake. They exposed a generation of children to one of the most toxic substances on the planet at levels that greatly exceeded safety levels in adults. And they administered it when they were most vulnerable. The magnitude of this mistake may explain the enormous efforts to divert attention from the true cause of autism. Geneticist Mark Geier, M.D., Ph.D., the President of The Genetic Centers of America refers to mercury in vaccines as "...the worst mistake that's been made in the history of medicine."

While the US CDC was backpedaling to cover up this catastrophic mistake, they misrepresented the findings of a study performed on monkeys by Thomas Burbacher. Burbacher compared the type of mercury injected in vaccinations with an oral form, which simulated eating contaminated fish. His results showed that the injectable type of mercury left the blood stream very rapidly (seven days) while the oral mercury took much longer (20–30 days). The US CDC used this data to publicly announce that the mercury contained in vaccinations was much safer than that consumed by eating fish. What they failed to mention is that the injected mercury that was cleared so rapidly from the bloodstream was not eliminated from the body. Rather, it became lodged in the brain where it has been known to remain for more than 20 years.[23]

Testimony from the Subcommittee on Human Rights and Wellness states that mercury, "... used as a preservative in vaccines is likely related to the autism epidemic. This epidemic in all probability may have been prevented or curtailed had the FDA not been asleep at the switch regarding injected [mercury] and the sharp rise of infant exposure to this known neurotoxin. Our public health agencies' failure to act is indicative of institutional malfeasance for self-protection and misplaced protectionism of the pharmaceutical industry."[24]

And yet, the debate continues. Parents are still told that vaccines are not to blame for the autism epidemic. Parents are fighting to increase awareness. How is it that I knew enough not to eat tuna fish more than a few times a month while pregnant, but had no idea that toxic levels of mercury could be in my daughter's shots? I wish I had heard the message from these parents several years ago. And yet these selfless parents have been labeled as hysterical or crazy. These parents are not hysterical; they are exhausted, tired of the run around, and just want justice. Most of these parents aren't even fighting for their own children who have already been affected. They are fighting to protect others from the same fate. They should be placed on pedestals, not blasted with contempt.

> **"...you can make a difference. Almost every significant advance that has ever happened for autism has ultimately been the result of the efforts of parents. This is not a disease that is going to be cured from the top down. It's going to be cured from the bottom up."**
> **-Bryan Jepson, M.D.**

Mercury: It's Still In There

> **"A major cause of the Roman Empire's decline after six centuries of world dominance, was its replacement of stone aqueducts by lead pipes for the transport and supply of drinking water. Roman engineers, the best in the world, turned their fellow citizens into cripples. Today our own "best and brightest," with the best of intentions, achieve the same end through childhood vaccination programs yielding the modern scourges of hyperactivity, learning disabilities, autism, appetite disorders, and impulsive violence."**
> **-Harris Coulter**

166

The good news is that our children are no longer receiving massive doses of mercury in their vaccinations. The bad news is that some vaccinations still contain the poison. The flu shot (if drawn from a multi-dose vial), tetanus shot, meningitis vaccine, and diphtheria and tetanus toxoids for pediatric use (but not the DTaP) may still contain mercury. Additionally, trace amounts of mercury may be present in mercury-free vaccines due to manufacturing processes.

As developed nations have eliminated mercury from the majority of their vaccines, the pharmaceutical industry has begun to exploit new markets by shipping it overseas to developing nations. For example, an aggressive pediatric marketing campaign was begun in China. In 2004, a few years after the mercury-laden vaccinations began to be administered, the official Chinese news agency reported that cases of autism had skyrocketed from nearly nothing to about 1.8 million children.[25]

Natural Immunity versus Artificial Immunizations

In the wake of this major vaccination debacle, we are continually bombarded with more and more vaccines. How can we weigh the risks and benefits of each vaccination when it can take generations for the adverse reactions to become apparent? We are now mandated to "protect" our children from chicken pox, a former rite of passage, and other not so devastating diseases.

A vaccination for a sexually transmitted disease that may lead to cervical cancer has now surfaced. Concerned physicians believe that mandating such a vaccine is the only way to protect low socioeconomic children from contracting the virus and future cervical cancer. While this cause is certainly noble, cervical cancer is rarely deadly and many people harbor the virus without developing cancer. How can anyone ethically force an entire generation of young girls to be exposed to a substance whose long-term effects are unknown when the benefits of the vaccine are probably minimal? Besides, history has shown that if there is a safety issue it will likely be hidden from us.

Even if vaccines are free of mercury and other toxins, we are not yet aware of the extent that they affect the immune system—our greatest ally in the fight to remain healthy. It is simply bad medicine to tinker with the normal function of the body in circumstances that are not of dire urgency. Obviously, the validity of vaccination against smallpox when it was once an epidemic is not in question, because the benefits clearly outweighed the detriments.

> **Cervical Cancer Vaccine:** A study published in the *New England Journal of Medicine* (NEJM) in June of 2007 showed that the cervical cancer vaccine was only 17 percent effective in reducing cervical cancer in girls in the general population, raising serious concerns regarding its effectiveness. More troublesome are the number of bad reactions that have already been reported to the FDA's Vaccine Adverse Event Reporting System (VAERS), including the deaths of three young girls.[26]

Regarding less dire medical conditions, we should focus on strengthening natural immunity rather than providing artificial immunizations. I doubt the push for more vaccines will ever end given the profits drug companies stand to make once their product is mandated by the government. We must demand that the benefits of vaccinations outweigh their risks. Long-term safety and effectiveness studies must be performed by independent researchers with no conflicts of interest *before* the product is mandated for use.

Avoiding Vaccinations

> **"Mandatory vaccine programs are 'A violation of the Nuremberg Code in that they force individuals to have medical treatment against their will or to participate in the functional equivalent of a vast experiment without fully informed consent.'"**
> **- Dr. Jane Orient, M.D., in a statement issued by the Association of American Physicians & Surgeons for the purpose of testimony before the Committee on Government Reform**

Because of the problems described earlier in this chapter, many parents have elected not to vaccinate their children. Children who are not vaccinated have been denied access to daycare, school, and federally funded assistance programs. Adults may be unable to apply for certain jobs. And so, a subculture of home-schooled, unvaccinated children has arisen.

Other Toxic Exposures
Vaccinations are not the only means of mercury exposure. Mercury is a component of silver dental fillings. These were once believed to be inert, but are now believed to leach mercury into the body. This is especially worrisome for pregnant women and young children who are still developing.

Mercury contamination of fish has been well publicized, resulting in avoidance of certain species and reduction in the quantity of fish that is advisable to consume. The EPA believes that 0.1 micrograms of mercury per kg of body weight per day is the amount of mercury a person can be exposed to on a daily basis over a lifetime without appreciable risk. The FDA has determined seafood with less than 1 part per million of mercury to be acceptable, but does not take action when fish sold at the grocery store or in restaurants exceeds this level.[27] One study found that 68 percent of swordfish samples were above the FDA Action Level and 16 percent were twice the FDA's Action Level.[28]

Mercury is also present in air pollution. According to the US Environmental Protection Agency, 144 tons of mercury was deposited in the US in 2001.[29] Visit **www.cleantheair.org** to identify where the coal-fired powerplants are located in your state and how much mercury they are emitting. One study performed in Rhode Island determined that autism was as prevalent in rural areas as in urban areas. However, when the researcher delved deeper into the history of each autistic family, she discovered that nearly all cases of autism occurred in children whose mothers resided in urban centers while pregnant or while the afflicted children were young. The researcher attributes this to exposure to urban air pollution during crucial stages of development.[30]

When all of these routes of exposure are considered together, children are exposed to an enormous toxic load. A 2004 study of umbilical cords revealed that every year 630,000 US infants are exposed to dangerous levels of mercury while still in the womb.[31] The public outcry from this study has resulted in improved efforts to reduce or eliminate exposure to mercury. These efforts include limiting mercury-contaminated fish consumption in pregnancy and monitoring mercury emissions from industry. In 2005 the EPA issued the Clean Air Mercury Rule to regulate mercury emissions from industrial plants. This is the first time mercury emissions from powerplants have ever been regulated in the US.

Mercury is not the only contaminant that causes developmental delays. Exposure to other toxins, such as aluminum, nickel or lead also contributes to the toxic burden that may lead to developmental problems. Researchers from the Harvard School of Public Health and the Mount Sinai School of Medicine have identified 202 industrial chemicals that share the ability to harm the human brain. Exposure to these chemicals in the womb or early childhood can lead to abnormal brain development and may explain the escalating rates of autism and attention deficit disorder. Sadly, 200 of these 202 brain toxins are not currently regulated. Moreover, the researchers are aware of more than 1,000 additional chemicals that have displayed similar toxicity problems in the brains of animals. It is reasonable to assume that many of these chemicals have the capacity to harm the human brain as well.[32]

While appallingly little is known about the long-term effects of all these toxins, much has been learned by exposing virtually every child born in an industrialized nation between 1960 and 1980 to a now well known brain toxin: lead. Lead is believed to have reduced IQ rates, shortened attention spans, impaired motor coordination, and increased aggressiveness in exposed children. Lead has also been linked to increased rates of developing Parkinson's disease and other nervous system disorders later in life. Fortunately, much effort has been directed at reducing or eliminating exposure to lead.

Diagnosing Mercury Toxicity

Porphyrins are precursors in the production of heme, which is what carries oxygen to the cells via the hemoglobin. Heavy metals, such as mercury, block the production of heme. Because heme is no longer being made, the ingredients used to assemble it, the porphyrins, begin to stack up. Eventually they spill over into the urine where they can be measured. There are many different porphyrins and the urine concentrations of these porphyrins will differ, based on which heavy metals are causing toxicity. One of these porphyrins, coproporphyrin, has been found to be elevated in the urine of children with autism compared to those without. Excess porphyrins may also be linked to seizure disorders. Porphyrin levels have been successfully reduced to normal by the process of chelation, which is explained later in this chapter.[33]

Test for Mercury Toxicity: The specific pattern that identifies mercury toxicity may have been removed from urine porphyrin tests performed in the US. Ask your physician to email the laboratory in France that performs the test with the mercury pattern at: **contact@labbio.net**. They can then perform this test for you. A healthcare provider who has attended a Defeat Autism Now! (DAN!) conference may be most able to assist you. Their physician referral list is accessible from **www.autism.com** under "Defeat Autism Now! List of Clinicians".

Ignoring Treatment

> **"Today, for the first time in history, there are successfully treated autistic children—living, breathing, speaking autistic children—living among us and enjoying their lives. These mainstreamed children, who no longer carry the dreaded label 'autistic', owe their liberation to treatment modalities which were, and still are, ridiculed, reviled, and rejected by most of the recognized authorities in the educational and medical autism establishments."**
>
> **-Bernard Rimland, Ph.D., President, Autism Research Institute**

It is standard protocol to remove heavy metals through a process called chelation. This involves administering a substance that the metal can bind to, like a magnet, in order to coax it out of the brain and other tissues in order to be flushed out of the body. When a child is diagnosed with lead poisoning they are placed on a chelation program. Yet, autistic children are not offered this treatment approach by mainstream medicine. Why not? I imagine that dramatic recoveries through removal of mercury will only reinforce the obvious: mercury toxicity contributes to autism. The public outcry would be tremendous and costly.

Another problem in using chelation is that it is difficult to identify elevated mercury levels in autistic children. The reason for this is simple. They are unable to detoxify and excrete the mercury so it is not present in their urine or hair samples. It remains lodged in their delicate brains. These children must first be chelated in order to mobilize the mercury out of their brain and into their urine where it can be measured. A study by Bradstreet et al. confirmed this by finding mercury levels in the urine of autistic children that were six times higher than nonautistic children once the mercury was mobilized by chelation.[34]

Dr. Rashid Buttar, DO, Vice Chairman of the American Board of Clinical Metal Toxicologists, testified before the Subcommittee on Human Rights and Wellness, US Congress on May 6, 2004 regarding his successful treatment of autistic children. "It is the elimination of this 'spark', i.e. mercury, for which we now have an easy and effective solution. Along with some supportive therapies, autism and certain other neurodegenerative diseases can be fully and permanently reversed. This is not a theory, but rather a protocol that has already been clinically validated and the evidence is irrefutable."[35] According to Stephanie Cave, M.D., Author of *What Your Doctor May Not Tell You About Children's Vaccinations*, "The good news is that (autistic children) are responding well to the chelation treatment. The changes in neurological functioning are remarkable with each day of treatment."

In addition to chelation therapy, administering co-enzymes that support detoxification processes have been found helpful in healing autistic children.[36] Treatment appears to be most successful at younger ages, so time is of the essence.

Autism and the Rest of the Body

There is a lot more to autism than just a "brain effect." Autistic children frequently have severe digestive problems. They often suffer from "leaky guts," which allow common foods to become allergens and enable foreign pathogens to access the body. Frequently, treating their stomach ailments resolves many of their aberrant behaviors and other symptoms.

Because 70 percent of the immune system is located in the gut, impaired digestion can lead to abnormal immune function. While most scientists and physicians focus on only a portion of the body at a time, Martha Herbert, a pediatric neurologist at Harvard Medical School, recognizes that the abnormalities seen in autistic brains occur in conjunction with immune system and other abnormalities.

Environmental toxins may cause an imbalance in the immune system, which allows a myriad of disorders to develop over one's lifetime. If the toxins strike during crucial developmental stages, the damage may be permanent. Genetic differences in the ability to rid the body of toxins may mean the difference between those who become ill and those who do not. Playing into the hands of Charles Darwin's concept of survival of the fittest, the Industrial

Revolution may have inadvertently tilted the scales in favor of organisms with the strongest detoxification abilities.

The Childhood Autism Risks from Genetics and the Environment study is now underway. Early findings suggest that the immune systems of children with autism function at lower levels than other children.[37] This indicates a link between immune system dysfunction and autism.

Some researchers believe that autistic children have immune systems that are out of balance. Some children exhibit decreased immunity making them more susceptible to infections, allergies, and chronic inflammation. These children seem to be sick all the time. Other children have a hyper-immune state; their over-zealous immune system attacks itself leading to autoimmune disorders. Indeed, it has been observed that autistic children often have significant family histories of autoimmune disorders.[38]

What Can You Do?

As with any medical procedure or treatment, weigh the risks and benefits before making an informed decision about vaccinations. Although most of the mercury has now been removed from childhood vaccinations, you may wish to delay the administration of some or all of them until the child's immune system is developed and/or space them out over time so that your child's immune system can better handle them. Tell your doctor you are concerned about the number of vaccinations and ask their advice about receiving an alternate schedule. If you feel the benefits of the flu shot outweigh the risks, be sure it is administered from a single dose vial. If you are pregnant, ask your doctor if you may require the Rhogam shot; if so, demand that it be given out of a single dose vial.

Some indications that your child may be more vulnerable to the negative effects of vaccinations include the following:

☐ If autoimmune disorders such as rheumatoid arthritis, lupus, or multiple sclerosis run in your family

☐ If your child began acting "funny" or developed a negative reaction after a previous round of vaccinations

☐ If another child in your family has autism or Asperger's syndrome

☐ If your child exhibits signs of attention deficit or hyperactivity

☐ If your child does not eat a wholesome diet that contains the nutrients needed to assist with the body's natural ability to detoxify

☐   If your child is sick and their immune system is concentrating on another task, such as fighting off a cold or other illness

If you wish to delay or reconsider vaccination, discuss this with a knowledgeable doctor, preferably one who has attended a Defeat Autism Now! (DAN!) conference (**www.autism.com**).

Chapter 20

*D*ental Fillings

According to Dietrich Klinghardt M.D., PhD, "Eighty percent of patients' health problems can be partially traced to the mouth." Although virtually all substances utilized by dentists have known toxicities, mercury is considered the greatest health threat of them all.

Mercury, a component of silver dental fillings, is a heavy metal and a potent nervous system toxin. Heavy metals have been dubbed the "21st century plague" because of widespread exposure and their devastating health effects. These effects are as numerous as they are diverse.

Mercury interferes with proper functioning of hemoglobin, which is needed to transport oxygen to cells, and with the production of ATP, which is crucial in manufacturing energy. These two mechanisms allow tiny, seemingly insignificant, doses of mercury to poison virtually every bodily function. Mercury is also capable of binding to random cells in the body, making them appear foreign to the immune system, so that it begins attacking itself. Genetic susceptibilities determine which autoimmune disorders may result once mercury confuses the immune system into destroying what were once normal body cells. Mercury also reduces the concentration of glutathione, which is a major detoxifier, leading to increased susceptibility to illness from other toxic exposures.

These effects lead to a multitude of seemingly unrelated symptoms and disorders. People exposed to mercury may develop neurological symptoms or diseases such as depression, Alzheimer's disease, Parkinson's disease, MSclerosis, MS, Lou Gehrig's disease, etc. They may also suffer from anxiety, forgetfulness, irritability, sleep disturbances, mood swings, low body temperature, cold hands or feet, swelling , excessive sweating, osteoporosis, thyroid or adrenal dysfunction, decreased fertility, anemia, irregular heartbeat, unexplained chest pain, abnormal blood pressure, elevated cholesterol, asthma, colitis, constipation, diarrhea, ulcers, food sensitivities, bloating, heartburn, belching, gas, nausea, headaches, dizziness, muscle twitching, seizures, confusion or brain fog, ringing in the ears, tremors, metallic taste in the mouth, bleeding gums, canker sores, sore throat, acne, skin rash, hair loss, and on and on.

Many people have been led to believe that once mercury is placed in the mouth in the form of silver dental fillings (called amalgams in the dental community), that the mercury remains tucked safely away inside the cavity. Scientists have unequivocally proven that this is not true. People with mercury fillings exhaled an average 15-fold increase in mercury vapor than those without.[1] This vapor is absorbed into the bloodstream where it gains access to all cells. A study on human cadavers revealed that those with mercury fillings had significantly higher amounts of mercury in their kidneys and brains than those without the fillings.[2]

Toxic mercury can be passed from a pregnant or nursing mother to her unborn or young child by crossing the placenta and via the breast milk.[3] The US EPA considers 0.1 micrograms per kilogram per day as the safety threshold of mercury to protect unborn children from brain damage. Each mercury filling releases about 10 micrograms of mercury into the body daily.[4] This means that any woman under 100 kg (220 pounds) would be exposing her unborn child to toxic mercury doses if she had even one mercury filling in her mouth. Because of this, California has mandated that signs be visible in dental offices alerting patients of the risk of birth defects associated with mercury fillings in the mouths of mothers-to-be.

The EPA and the National Academy of Sciences have declared that a large percentage of American women have mercury levels high enough to cause potential neurological damage to their unborn children. A survey conducted by the US CDC indicates that more than 10 percent of women of reproductive age in the US have blood mercury levels that may increase the risk of impaired brain development in their children.[5] Indeed, the effect has already been observed: the US CDC has concluded that 1 in 6 American children have a neurodevelopmental disorder.

Yet, I was not aware of the dangers of mercury fillings. I recall specifically asking my dentist whether silver fillings were bad for health and received a sunny reassurance that they were completely safe. I went on to have the last of nearly 20 silver fillings placed just before becoming pregnant. While researching this book I began to wonder why my dentist had falsely reassured me. Initially I believed that dental programs must omit the dangers of mercury fillings from the curriculum in much the same way as my physician assistant training omitted the dangers of vaccinations.

However, a telephone conversation with Dr. Hal Huggins, D.D.S., M.S., an expert in mercury removal and utilizing dental substances that are compatible with individual immune systems, opened my eyes to the scandalous behavior of the American Dental Association (ADA), who happen to hold the patent on mercury fillings.

Until a recent Congressional Committee found that the FDA had failed to protect the public from the danger of mercury in dentistry, the ADA Code of Ethics once punished dentists who advised their patients that mercury might be dangerous. Many of these well-meaning dentists lost their license to practice dentistry because they warned their patients of mercury's inherent risks.[6]

In response to the Congressional Committee's findings, the ADA recently distributed a letter to dentists advising them to warn women of the dangers of mercury fillings to the unborn fetus. Although this action was intended to protect themselves by deflecting potential lawsuits from the ADA to individual dentists, the ADA's action marks a turning point in the battle to protect people from the dangers of mercury in dental fillings. According to Dr. Hal Huggins, the actions undertaken by the ADA regarding mercury fillings is not a conspiracy theory, but a conspiracy reality. Fortunately, the conspiracy is now out in the open allowing the opportunity to finally eliminate the use of mercury in dentistry.[7]

If you or a loved one suffers from symptoms that cannot be resolved by conventional medicine, consider the removal of silver fillings. However, don't rush right out and get the fillings removed without researching the safest course of action. When mercury is removed from the teeth, the body must be prepared to eliminate the toxic metal quickly so that it is not deposited in the brain or other vital organs. Because of the redistribution of the toxin, 63 percent of people who have mercury fillings removed end up with a disease they did not suffer with prior to its removal. For this reason, mercury fillings must be removed in a cautious manner by a dentist trained to remove them safely.[8]

This doctor should also perform a blood test to determine which alternate filling type is most compatible with your particular immune system. All dental fillings contain some inherently hazardous materials, but each individual is able to handle certain substances better than others. To find a dentist that has been trained by Dr. Huggins and his team to safely remove mercury fillings, call 1-866-948-4638. For more information read *It's All in Your Head*, by Dr. Hal Huggins.

*T*riumph Over Toxins

**"Hope for the earth lies not with leaders but in your
own heart and soul. If you decide to save the earth, it
will be saved."**
                    **–Helen Caldicott, Founder of Physicians for
                    Social Responsibility**

*The previous section unveiled a multitude of ways to reduce our
chemical exposure. However, complete avoidance of toxic chemicals
is not going to be possible in our lifetime. In fact, many toxic
chemicals are persistent and will continue to afflict future
generations. While such news is certainly disheartening, this does
not necessarily mean we are sentenced to a lifetime of illness. The
human body has been designed to heal itself; strengthening our
ability to detoxify will provide the best chance for good health.*

Chapter 21

An Apple a Day

"Let food be your medicine."
–Hippocrates, the Father of Medicine

We are each born with an arsenal of defenses to protect us from becoming sick. If these defenses are strong we stand a better chance of remaining well despite the onslaught of toxic exposures. Therefore, supporting the immune system and preventing its imbalance or weakness is fundamental in preserving health.

Supporting the immune system can be accomplished by insuring proper nutrition, a healthy balance of rest and exercise, adequate social support, and other lifestyle factors. Preventing the immune system from being overwrought can be accomplished by avoiding external toxins, foreign invaders, trauma, and other stressors.

According to the Centers for Disease Control, "Virtually all human diseases result from the interaction of genetic susceptibilities and modifiable environmental factors". This means that by eating a healthy, whole-food diet along with individualized nutritional supplementation, exercising, maintaining a healthy weight, and avoiding toxins, we can alter the way our genes are expressed. In other words, we can overcome inherited tendencies toward diseases by adopting a healthier lifestyle.

"To fight a disease after it has occurred is like digging a well when one is thirsty or forging a weapon once a war has begun."
–The Yellow Emperor's Classic of Internal Medicine.
Nei Ching. Circa 1,000 BC.

What To Enjoy
When we think of a diet, let's focus on what we should be eating rather than what we should not. We are so preoccupied by what we can't put in our mouths that eating has become a major source of stress. According to Dr. Susan Lord, director of Food as Medicine course, "Food is the solution, not the problem." By

selecting fresh, natural products rather than processed foods or those that contain additives, we will supply our bodies with nutrients vital for health. Once we have eaten enough servings of tasty, nutrient rich, beneficial foods, we will have little room left for junk.

Nature's Anti-inflammatory

Foods rich in omega-6 fatty acids promote inflammation whereas those rich in omega-3 fatty acids suppress inflammation. A balance between the two is vital. The Standard American Diet (with the appropriate acronym of SAD) provides about a 27:1 ratio of omega-6 fatty acids to omega-3 fatty acids. Optimal health requires a ratio closer to 2:1 or 3:1. To improve your ratio, try incorporating more of the following into your diet: fish that is not farmed, animal products that are grain fed, and/or fish oil (DHA/EPA) supplements that are certified to be free of toxins.

Animals that are grass-fed have a higher concentration of healthy omega-3 fatty acids than their counterparts fed a traditional agribusiness diet. The eggs laid by such grain fed animals are also high in omega-3 fatty acids while others are not. Because of their diet, farmed fish have a lower percentage of omega-3 fatty acids than their wild counterparts.

Foods that combat inflammation include those that are rich in omega-3 fatty acids, such as cold water, wild-caught fish. Try to avoid fish with high mercury content and PCBs by selecting fish that are lower on the food chain and remove the skin and fat which is where PCBs accumulate. Fish higher up on the food chain are likely to contain the highest levels of mercury and other toxins because they accumulate in fat and are more concentrated as they pass up the food chain. Wild salmon, tilapia, herring, and sardines are examples of good choices.

Contact your state or local health department for more information on which fish are safe to eat and limit your intake to the recommended guidelines. This is especially important in pregnant woman because mercury causes neurological damage to the fetus and PCBs have been linked to deficits in intelligence and behavioral disorders in offspring.

Other sources of healthy omega-3 fatty acids include nuts and seeds, which should be added to your diet. Keep them refrigerated and try to buy organic nuts that are still in their shells, unsalted, and unroasted.

Anti-Inflammatory Diet: Patients suffering from rheumatoid arthritis had a 14 percent decrease in joint tenderness and swelling when following an anti-inflammatory diet compared to those who ate a Standard American Diet. If they incorporated fish oil supplements, they had a 31 percent reduction in such symptoms. Patients following a Mediterranean diet, whose recommendations are similar to those above, had more than a 70 percent reduction of heart attacks and death. That is an astounding accomplishment. In a French study, seniors who consumed an anti-inflammatory diet consisting of fish at least once a week were less likely to develop Alzheimer's disease.

A Rainbow a Day

Eating a rainbow of colorful fruits and vegetables is a wonderful suggestion made by Dr. Nicholas Perricone, author of the *Perricone Promise*, which is a wonderful resource for healthy eating. Most natural healing experts recommend nine half-cup servings of fruits and vegetables a day. (This should keep you busy and away from the chips!)

Nutrition experts believe that five servings of fruits and vegetables are insufficient to supply the nutrients needed for optimum health. Indeed, the recommended daily allowances are based on quantities of nutrients needed to avoid overt diseases such as scurvy, not for the prevention of chronic diseases or preservation of optimal health. It is a better idea to try to incorporate 10 servings a day of a rainbow of foods. These foods supply a host of disease fighting compounds known as phytonutrients as well as vitamins and minerals.[1]

Red foods (i.e. apples, beets, cherries, grapes, tomatoes, and strawberries), orange foods (i.e. apricots, carrots, peaches, and squash), yellow foods (i.e. bananas, cauliflower, corn, pears, garlic, and onions), and blue/violet foods (i.e. blueberries, cabbage, plums, eggplant, and grapes) provide Vitamins A and C. Green foods (e.g. kiwi, broccoli, cucumbers, parsley, peas, spinach, and leafy vegetables) supply Vitamins A, B, C, and E. Brown/gold foods (e.g. whole grains, oatmeal, beans, figs, raisins, and dates) provide Vitamins B and E. Vitamin D is derived from sun exposure or supplementation.

One serving is equivalent to a handful of nuts, ¼ cup dried fruit, ½ cup fresh fruit or vegetables, 1 slice whole grain bread, ½ cup oatmeal, and ½ cup legumes or green leaves. Visit

www.Whfoods.org to learn more about the world's healthiest foods.

Organic and Locally Grown

Choose organic produce whenever possible to avoid dangerous pesticide residues. Although these toxins are absorbed into the produce, scrubbing and peeling will help if you must buy conventional produce. If cost is a factor, try growing your own, joining or starting a community garden or co-op, or having a container garden on a balcony or windowsill. Some urban schools have integrated a school garden into the curriculum. Consider bringing a similar program to your school district. Check out **www.kidsgardening.com** for resources or to apply for a grant.

Locally grown produce is another great option. Because such food does not need to endure long shipping times, it is picked at its peak and contains more nutrients. Such produce is often cheaper than certified organic produce and requires fewer preservatives to make it to market. Supporting local farmers who grow their food in a sustainable, chemical-free manner is good for you as well as the planet. Visit your local farmer's market today. If necessary, start one in your community.

When to Splurge on Organic: The US Department of Agriculture has determined that certain fruits and vegetables are heavily laden with pesticides even after washing. The Environmental Working Group (EWG) recommends that such produce never be purchased in conventional form and are worth the extra expense of buying their organic counterparts. Splurge on organic whenever buying the following: apples, cherries, imported grapes, nectarines, peaches, pears, raspberries, strawberries, bell peppers, celery, potatoes, and spinach. Along with the produce listed above, Consumer Reports listed green beans and winter squash as having higher toxicity scores than other fruits and vegetables. On the other hand, the following fruits and vegetables generally do not contain pesticide residue and can be purchased conventionally if you are on a tight budget: bananas, kiwi, mangos, papaya, pineapples, asparagus, avocado, broccoli, cauliflower, onions, and peas. Go to **www.foodnews.org** to look for updates or to view the complete list. They also have a free pocket guide to take with you when you shop.

Healthier Meat

Whenever possible, choose free-range, grass-fed meat products that have not been given growth hormones or antibiotics. Remove the fat from meats as many toxins accumulate there. Current methods of raising animals for food involve poor nutrition, the need for antibiotics to protect these weaker animals from infection, and the use of growth hormones. These meats contain a higher percentage of inflaming omega-6 fatty acids than their less stressed cousins who are raised on a healthful diet in a more humane manner.

Affording Organic: I assumed, as I imagine many of us do, that switching to organic food and other healthier alternatives would seriously strain our budget, but I was pleasantly surprised to find the reverse to be true. While our budget for food increased astronomically, we saved a similar amount of money by eating out much less frequently. I just couldn't stomach eating in restaurants or fast food establishments once I knew what was in the food. By adopting a healthier lifestyle, we inadvertently went on a debt diet. There is no stronger incentive to stop shopping than the thought that practically every item sold commercially in some manner harms my daughter. I simply don't need to buy as much.

Organic meat can be expensive, so purchase cheap organic beans to counteract this hefty blow to your grocery bill. If you cannot afford the more expensive meat, stick with the beans. They are much healthier than standard American meat. I often increase the nutrients in my meals while reducing their cost by blending canned beans (always rinse them first to remove any harmful residue from the plastic coating of the can) and adding them to ground beef before cooking. My family doesn't even know they are in there!

Another benefit to both your health and your wallet stems from incorporating more meat and dairy-free meals into your weekly routine. Visit the Physicians Committee for Responsible Medicine website (**www.pcrm.org**) to learn more about the negative health effects of meat and dairy and the truth about calcium.

High Fiber

Fiber speeds the transit of toxins out of the digestive tract; therefore, it is important for detoxification. Fiber binds toxins, such as excess estrogen, pesticides, mercury, etc., and carries them out of the body. A diet high in plant products, such as unprocessed beans, vegetables, fruits, and whole grains will increase fiber consumption and decrease digestive disorders, colon cancer, breast cancer, stomach cancer, heart disease, diabetes, and other illnesses.[2]

Preserving Nutrients

The way that food is prepared is as important as the choices we make. One study showed that overcooked broccoli from a hospital cafeteria was devoid of its beneficial nutrients. The best way to prepare vegetables is to sauté them in olive oil or to incorporate them into soups, stews, or chilies so that the nutrients aren't discarded with the water.

Cooking at high temperatures can cause the formation of free radicals, which spark the disease process. To avoid "charring" food, keep the cooking temperature below 350 degrees. Although olive oil is an excellent choice for sautéing food, be sure to avoid high temperatures. When frying or cooking at high temperatures, use only palm or coconut oils, which can withstand these high temperatures without releasing dangerous free radicals.

Eggs are one example of a food that requires careful preparation to avoid destruction of its nutrients. Eggs that are poached or hard-boiled are preferable to other cooking methods.

Rancid Oils: If the oil starts so smoke while you are cooking, dangerous free radicals are being formed. It is best to discard the oil and start over at a lower temperature.

Herbs and Spices

Herbs are not regulated by the US FDA. Your best bet for a safe product is to buy one labeled with a seal of approval from the United States Pharmacopeia (USP) or Consumerlab.com (CL). Check out www.consumerlab.com to research specific brands before you buy.

The Green Pharmacy by James A. Duke is a great resource for choosing herbs and supplements. One example of a healthful spice is turmeric, which is one of the curry spices and contains a powerful anti-inflammatory known as curcumin. According to a 2006 study in the Journal of Alzheimer's Disease, curcumin can reduce the characteristic brain plaques in Alzheimer's disease. A 2006 Johns Hopkins study showed that it also reduced the number of precancerous colon polyps by 60 percent.

Getting Started

Several great books regarding healthful diets are listed in Appendix I. The World's Healthiest Foods website (**www.Whfoods.org**) is a great resource for recipes, shopping lists, and information about healthy eating. If you need help motivating your children to eat right, try the Nutrition Detectives Program by Dr. David Katz. (**www.davidkatzmd.com**).

Chapter 22

*D*etoxification

On September 11, 2001, terrorists deliberately crashed airplanes into the two colossal towers that once comprised the World Trade Center (WTC). Who could forget such a tragedy? A black cloud of jet fuel containing volatile organic compounds, such as benzene and hydrocarbons was emitted upon impact. The buildings themselves were pulverized into a fine powder that blanketed lower Manhattan.

The dust contained lead, PCBs, dioxin, asbestos, fiberglass, plastics, and other poisonous chemicals. The plume of toxic smoke traveled Southwest increasing respiratory complaints among residents in lower Manhattan and Brooklyn.[1] The rubble continued to emit toxic by-products as it burned for several months and as rescue workers and the clean-up crew manipulated the pile. The burning of PVC and plastic from the rubble released airborne toxins that measured thousands of times higher than the presumed safe exposure level. WTC rescue workers and residents were exposed to numerous toxins, many of which are known to accumulate in body tissues.

One of my family members, a New York City police officer who was stationed at Ground Zero immediately after the tragedy, was recently in the intensive care unit due to a weak heart. He also has an irregular heart rhythm, pneumonia, and inflammation of his lungs, which his doctors suspect is due to sarcoidosis. Sarcoidosis is a hot topic nowadays because numerous workers at Ground Zero, in the WTC rubble, are developing it.

Many rescue workers are now paying the price for their selfless acts of heroism. A study performed at Mount Sinai Hospital found that nearly 70 percent of WTC responders had a new or worsened respiratory symptom since working at Ground Zero. Many workers had decreased lung function that persisted as long as two-and-a-half years after the disaster.[2]

Thousands of once robust workers now suffer from a host of neurological problems such as headaches, short-term memory loss, and difficulty concentrating. In the absence of an appropriate disease to which to attribute these symptoms, they are said to have the "World Trade Center Flu." But it is not the flu. It is a host of symptoms caused by an unprecedented exposure to toxic fumes.

While respiratory problems are the obvious result of inhaling copious amounts of dust, soot, and smoke, it is only the tip of the iceberg. Once tiny particles of foreign material reach the small sacs in the lungs where oxygen exchange occurs, the toxins only have to cross one cell layer to gain access to the bloodstream. When toxins invade the bloodstream via the lungs they are not transported directly to the liver for filtration as is the case when toxins are ingested from the gut. This means the potential for harm is greater. These toxins may cause acute illnesses as they travel throughout the body. They may also lodge themselves in fatty tissue such as the brain where they accumulate with other toxins that have been lodged there and predispose to a host of chronic ailments.[3]

In the years that have passed since the 9/11 atrocity, the rate of rapidly growing cancers, such as lymphoma and other cancers of the blood, are higher in rescue workers than expected. Slow growing cancers and other health problems may not reveal themselves for many more years. The magnitude of chronic illnesses resulting from the WTC exposure may never be known. However, what is becoming evident is that the death toll from 9/11 continues to climb as many succumb to the toxic effects of chemicals emitted from the rubble.

Fortunately, a detoxification program supported by private donations has led to miraculous recoveries for many of these heroes. The results from this detoxification program are stellar. A study of the initial 500 participants in the program, comprised mostly of firefighters, showed complete or almost complete resolution of memory impairment, poor concentration, insomnia, depression, irritability, fatigue, and headaches. Improvements were also seen in breathing difficulties, cough, shortness of breath with exercise, skin disorders, joint and muscle pain, vision, hearing, or smelling impairment, impotence, and gastrointestinal problems.[4] The detoxification program also eliminated the need for medication in 82 percent of participants who had required medication at the onset of the program.[5]

The program works by mobilizing toxins from fat cells, directing them to routes of elimination, and increasing the functionality of elimination routes. Exercise and sauna use facilitate the migration of toxins out of body tissues via sweating. Vitamins and other supplements are incorporated to strengthen the body's natural filtration abilities. Adequate fluid intake is a must as are ample vegetables to insure regular bowel movements, another route of elimination. Sufficient sleep is also required during the intensive program.

The program has been established to be safe and effective in reducing toxic loads of PCBs, DDT, and other foreign substances.[6] The program has been successful in detoxifying workers involved in the cleanup after the nuclear disaster at Chernobyl and several industrial fires, including firefighters exposed to an exploding transformer full of toxic PCBs. A Vietnam veteran and Gulf war veterans have had their lives transformed by this program as well.[7]

WTC program participants can attest to the successful elimination of toxins. As the participants' towels absorbed their sweat, they turned all different colors of the rainbow, reflecting the properties of the different toxins they contained. When one of the first program participants was in the sauna, the towel that he used to wipe his sweat turned a bright shade of blue. When the towel was analyzed it was found to contain manganese, a component of structural steel. If it remains stored in the body, manganese is known to cause a Parkinson-like syndrome about 5–10 years after exposure.[8]

As a cardiology physician assistant I used to perform annual stress tests on firefighters. It was often easy to pick these "patients" out in the waiting room because they didn't look like the majority of my other patients. The firefighters were typically younger and more robust than the elderly cardiac patients I routinely saw. But looks are often deceiving. I was surprised to find that many of these younger men were failing their stress tests, an indication that they may have blockages in the arteries of their hearts, which could lead to heart attacks. I attributed this to their firehouse diet, despite protests that they had begun cooking healthy meals for one another.

It has taken me a decade to put two and two together. The high rate of heart disease I witnessed in these firefighters was most likely not a result of the risk factors described in my medical textbooks. After all, most of the American population eats a diet as poor as theirs and aren't nearly as physically active, so why should firefighters be suffering from more heart disease? It is more likely a result of inflammation induced by toxic exposures in their line of work. Perhaps firefighters should undergo routine detoxification as a precautionary measure given their routine exposure to toxic fumes.

Thanks to generous donations, the New York Rescue Workers Detoxification Program, which was co-founded by Tom Cruise, is providing free detoxification services to eligible WTC rescue workers. Affected workers can go to **www.nydetox.org** or call (212) 587-3961 for details.

Perhaps we should all undergo routine detoxification since it has already been established that each of us carries our own toxic load. L. Ron Hubbard's book, *Clear Body Clear Mind*, offers valuable advice on how to detoxify. More information is available at **www.detoxacademy.org.**

Chapter 23

A Call to Action

"It is better to light a single candle than to curse the darkness."

-Unknown

Several decades ago Rachel Carson, whose book, *Silent Spring,* is credited with initiating the modern environmental movement, told Congress, "I hope this committee will give attention to the right of the citizen to be secure in his own home against the intrusion of poisons applied by other persons. This should be one of the basic human rights."[1] Apparently Congress has not yet felt the need to provide us with this basic human right.

American companies marked the beginning of the 21st century by releasing more than 7 billion pounds of industrial chemicals into the air or water; chemicals that didn't even exist when the previous century was ushered in. It is no wonder that chronic illnesses have emerged as the 21st century plague, diseases of adulthood are now commonplace in young children, and cancer rates have soared from only 1 in 8,000 Americans in 1901 to nearly 1 of every 2 individuals![2] It is time we stopped hedging and acknowledge the obvious: Toxic chemicals are bad for health and health is getting bad. Dr. David Katz said it best, "If your foot catches on fire, you don't need a randomized clinical trial to fetch a pail of water."

Rather than wasting more time, money, and energy on research, let's do something about it. The solution is surprisingly simple. All we need to do is reclaim responsibility for our own health rather than relying on others. We have the power to make a profound impact on the degradation of our environment and our health. Read on for specific tips on how to do this.

Choose Products Wisely

> **"It is truly enough said that a corporation has no conscience; but a corporation of conscientious men is a corporation with a conscience."**
>
> **–Henry David Thoreau**

The bad news is that current policies tend to permit chemicals wherever economic benefits outweigh potential harm, even if that harm equates to a handful of children dying of leukemia in your neighborhood. The good news is that economics are based on supply and demand. This means that we, as consumers, can eliminate the economic benefits of harmful chemicals by simply refusing to purchase products that contain them.

By boycotting toxic chemicals we are sending the corporate world a message they can't ignore. To make sure this message is loud and clear we each need to be sure to spread the word. There is certainly strength in numbers and we need that strength now. There are many examples of consumerism driving dangerous products off the shelves. For example, when asbestos was found to be causing a form of lung cancer called mesothelioma, a drop in consumer demand forced manufacturers to look for alternatives.

Bigger is Not Always Better

> **"The multinational corporation is the most powerful institution of our time, dominating not only global economics, but politics and culture as well. The enormous influence of the corporation notwithstanding, the mechanisms of corporate control and the details of corporate abuses remain largely hidden from public perception."**
>
> **–Excerpt from the Mokhiber-Weissman Column on Corporate Power**

The WTC tragedy created fervor among Americans to buy American made products. Unfortunately, many greedy American corporations have harmed more Americans than terrorists have. If we truly want to honor the victims of the 9/11 tragedy, we should support ethically-run businesses rather than corporate predators.

191

For a list of the top 100 corporate predators of the 1990s, go to **http://www.corporatepredators.org/**.
Also, remember to support your local farmers. Doing so encourages more environmentally sound procedures, fewer pesticides, and puts money back in the hands of families rather than corporate predators.

Purchasing products only from conscientious corporations, local farmers, and small, family-owned local businesses restores power to the people. Shopping has the same effect on corporations as voting has on politicians. Without our money, or vote, the product will not remain on store shelves. For this reason, every dollar we spend should be spent with great care. Every seemingly small decision about how to run our households or businesses has major consequences. Shopping is a tremendous responsibility. Who knew?

Restore Accountability

In Venice, Italy, executives were charged with manslaughter for knowingly exposing their workers to toxic chemicals that led to their deaths and endangering the general public by polluting the local river. Meanwhile, Philip Morris' scientists, who knew of the addictive qualities of cigarettes, walked away free.

Perhaps things would change in America if unscrupulous executives were held accountable for the safety of their products and for the safety of their emissions and discharges. It is naïve to assume that these executives are unaware of the crimes their corporations are committing. It is time we held them accountable.

Invest Wisely

While purchasing healthy products allows us to vote with our spending money, investing in companies that reflect our own value system also allows us to vote with our savings. Many people are already catching on to the importance of supporting companies that are socially responsible. "Socially Responsible" mutual funds grew from $12 billion in 1995 to $178.7 billion in the US in 2005, far outpacing the overall growth of mutual funds.[3] Nearly 1 in 10 dollars is now invested in a socially responsible manner.

That is an enormous amount of money, and therefore, an enormous incentive for companies who want our money to do the right thing. But only if we demand that they do. We can accomplish this by simply converting our investments to companies that respect our health and the health of the environment. Changing our investment portfolios really can make a difference. In the 1980s, major positive changes took place in South Africa when

192

individuals avoided investing in companies that benefited from Apartheid.[4] When we purchase stock we become part owner of a company. Before investing, take a step back and think, "Is this a company I can be proud of?"

Check out **www.socialfunds.com** or **www.socialinvest.org** to learn how to invest in a socially conscious manner.

Business is *Not* Just Business

> **"Our scientific power has outrun our spiritual power. We have guided missiles and misguided men."**
> **–Dr. Martin Luther King Jr.**

The phrase "business is business" implies that personal morals should be checked at the door when one enters the workplace. Most Americans spend the majority of waking hours working. If we must detach ourselves from our souls in order to prosper at work, how can we feel good about ourselves? Is it any wonder that Americans are depressed? There is simply no way to feel good about ourselves when we make decisions (business or otherwise) that go against our ethical beliefs. You cannot have one set of values in your personal life and another set for business.

Aaron Feuerstein proved that "business is business" is neither universally accepted nor applied. When his textile plant burned to the ground in 1995, he paid each of his employees in full for the next three months despite the fact that there was no work for them to do. He then rebuilt the plant at its original site rather than opting to relocate to an area where he could exploit cheap labor. When asked why he made these "poor" business decisions he replied that it would be unconscionable to put his 3,000 employees on the streets and "deliver a death blow to the city" by moving the company elsewhere. Because of the rarity of such acts of kindness, he became a national hero.

You can be a hero too. In each of your decisions, consider the impact on others and act according to your conscience. You will be left with a sense of peace that you may not find by any other means. Everyday heroes like Aaron Feuerstein are extraordinary. We need more of them.[5]

> **"The significant problems we face cannot be solved at the same level of thinking we were at when we created them."**
> **–Albert Einstein**

Many of us may need to reevaluate our career choices. We must ask ourselves, is what I am doing bettering the world? Am I making, marketing, or selling a product or performing a service that is going to improve the well-being of others? Am I sure that the good of the product or service outweighs the toll it takes on the environment in order to perform, produce or distribute it? Am I using my talents and abilities in the greatest possible way? If the answer to any of the above is "no," then it is time to create a better product, service, or system, or do a little soul-searching to come up with a new life plan.

Inspiring Change: Kate Roberts was featured in the February 2007 edition of O Magazine as a "Woman with Heart." While vacationing in South Africa, she experienced an "aha moment." She decided she could no longer sell cigarettes and soda so she changed the direction of her life. She founded YouthAIDS, and reconnected with her soul. So can you!

Renew Our Priorities

The National Children's Study (NCS) was designed to follow 100,000 US children from early pregnancy to 21 years of age in order to evaluate the health effects of toxic chemicals on development.[6] Unfortunately, this study lost funding and will be terminated prematurely. The findings would likely have confirmed the link between toxins and premature illness and death in children. It likely would have forced regulatory changes to protect our children.

The allocation of funding reflects our priorities as a country. Why are we funding research for medical conditions that keep older Americans living longer at the expense of studies that protect the lives and well-being of our children?

One Step Forward, Two Steps Back

> **The parable of the three blind men and the elephant: The first blind man feels the trunk and says, "This is a snake." The second blind man feels the elephant's leg and says, "This is a tree." The third blind man feels the elephant's tail and says, "This is a rope." Isn't it time we see the big picture?**

194

As the toxicity of chlorine has gained publicity, many water utilities have begun switching to alternate chemicals or mixtures of disinfectants. While eliminating the use of chlorine is certainly desirable, we must be sure we are not replacing a known toxin for one that has no reported toxicity simply because it is new and unstudied. We may be setting ourselves up for more harm than good.

In our quest to reduce our dependence upon petroleum products, the use of ethanol (alcohol) as an alternate fuel source is gaining popularity. The problem with using ethanol is that a toxic additive, methanol, is added to prevent it from being heavily taxed as liquor. Methanol makes the ethanol poisonous so that it cannot be consumed as an alcoholic beverage, thereby obviating the liquor tax. Inhaling methanol gas is toxic to humans and can lead to blindness or death. It is particularly toxic to pregnant women who are often deficient in folic acid, which helps to detoxify it. It is predicted that methanol contamination would increase significantly if we were to switch fuel sources.

Another problem with methanol is that it rapidly dissolves in water. This means that in the event of an accidental fuel spill, there will be no way to remove the toxin from the water. Essentially, the entire water body will become contaminated as there will be no "scum" to float to the top for removal as in the Exxon Valdez spill.

Another example is the push to use fluorescent light bulbs, which contain mercury. While energy efficiency is desirable, placing more toxic mercury in landfills is certainly not.

The bottom line is that while searching for alternatives to toxic products, we need to be cognizant of the fact that alternatives may one day be found to be more harmful. Choosing natural products rather than alternate chemicals is preferable whenever possible.

Support the Precautionary Principle

Chemicals are presently considered innocent until proven guilty. Despite the lack of prior consent or even the knowledge of those exposed, the chemical industry is allowed to expose millions of people, including children, to their products without ensuring their safety. If oversight agencies adopt the Precautionary Principle, which states that chemicals have to be proven safe *before* being placed on the market, this would change. Because this principle would interfere with profits, there is strong opposition to it. Let your legislators know that you expect them to act in the best interests of the people rather than chemical company pocketbooks.

"Sometimes the questions are complicated and the answers are simple."

–Dr. Seuss

We Must Save Ourselves

To regain our right to a healthy environment in which to raise healthy children we must rely on our families, friends, neighbors, communities, and most importantly, ourselves. Our children's health is more important than the conveniences of modern life.

I believe we can learn to do without the products that are manufactured by corporations who willingly harm our planet and our health. I believe we can convert our investments to funds that only invest in socially responsible companies. I believe we can encourage each other to endure a few inconveniences as we learn new ways of doing things. I believe we will demand that our children have the right to be born chemically free and the right to achieve their full potential. I believe that we will successfully spread the word by discussing these issues at Book Clubs, Mom's Clubs, Parent Teacher Association (PTA) meetings, civic group meetings such as the Rotary Club, Town Hall Meetings, business meetings, homeowner's association meetings, and anywhere else we gather.

As we work together toward our common goal, let us not judge one another. Each of us has unique abilities, disabilities, ambitions, and perceptions. Some of us are not ready to hear this message and some who have heard are not yet ready or able to act. Remember that everything appears different when our perspective changes. Let's not look upon our neighbors who appear wealthier and cast judgment upon their purchasing habits. In the eyes of street children from third world countries, we all have too much. Each one of us is wealthy beyond their wildest dreams. Concerning ourselves with others only distracts us from completing the task at hand.

A close friend of mine once shared with me a belief passed down through his family that guided each and every decision he made. He said, "In every thing you do or neglect to do, consider what the world would be like if everyone else did the same." That statement had a profound effect on me. It changed the way I thought about small, seemingly insignificant decisions, such as what to do with a candy wrapper while walking down a street with no garbage cans. While throwing an empty wrapper onto the street may seem insignificant, what would the world be like if it was strewn with everyone's trash?

The same is true with making great strides. Can you imagine what the world would be like if each of us refused to purchase foods laced with pesticides? There would no longer be a reason to manufacture pesticides. Mother Teresa once said, "We can't do great things, only small things with great love." These small things do add up. The next chapter will provide you with a 10-Step Action Plan so you can get started.

Chapter 24

*1*0-Step Action Plan

"All that is necessary for evil to prevail is for good men to do nothing."

-Edmund Burke

1. **Find Out Who is Making You Sick**

   a. Visit **http://www.scorecard.org**, type in your zipcode, and find out who is polluting your community, what they are releasing into your air and water, and what health problems the pollutants cause. Organize community members to discuss alternatives and solutions with the spokesperson for the worst polluters; their name and contact number are listed as well.

   b. Check out **www.bucketbrigade.net** to learn how to collect your own air quality data. Dozens of other communities have used this method to improve pollution and increase enforcement of environmental regulations.

2. **Select a Water Purification System**

   a. First, find out what you are up against by calling your local water company and requesting the Consumer Confidence Report.

   b. Then go to **http://www.ewg.org/tapwater/yourwater/index.php** to discover which unregulated contaminants you should be concerned about.

   c. Armed with this information, you can then look up each contaminant at **http://www.nsf.org** to find the "Standard" number that will be listed on water purifiers that are certified to remove the particular chemical.

   d. Then go to the Products page at **http://www.nsf.org** and select a product that meets these "Standards". If you need help, there is a phone number listed on their site.

  e. Bottle your own water to take on trips by refilling glass jars or stainless steel bottles. If you must purchase bottled water on occasion, check out **http://www.nrdc.org/water** to choose a brand that is relatively pure.

3. **Eliminate Toxic Food**
  a. Grow your own food in window boxes or a home or community garden
  b. Choose organic products, preferably from small, environmentally-friendly companies, whenever possible.
  c. Wash thoroughly and peel all non-organic produce.
  d. Avoid conventional apples, cherries, imported grapes, nectarines, peaches, pears, raspberries, strawberries, bell peppers, celery, potatoes, spinach, green beans, and winter squash.
  e. If you are on a tight budget, it's relatively safe to choose the following conventional items: bananas, kiwi, mangos, papaya, pineapples, asparagus, avocado, broccoli, cauliflower, onions, and peas. Go to **www.foodnews.org** to make sure this list is up-to-date.
  f. Find growth hormone-free dairy by searching the website of the Organic Consumers Association at **www.organicconsumers.org.**
  g. Find hormone-free beef as well as healthier poultry, eggs, etc., in your area at **http://www.eatwellguide.org**. This is also a great resource for travelers. Simply type in the zipcode where you are heading to locate healthier restaurants, farms, stores, etc.
  h. Moms, dads, grandparents and others are welcome to join the holistic moms' network (**http://www.holisticmoms.org**) where you can learn where healthier food is purchased in your neighborhood.

199

i.   Reduce consumption of processed foods. Avoid artificial sweeteners and "diet"

j.   products, nitrites in cured meats and many deli products, food colorings, and preservatives such as BHA, BHT.

k.   Look up ingredients you are not sure of at **http://www.cspinet.org/reports/chemcuisine.htm**

l.   Never microwave in plastic containers or wraps. Limit use of plastic, but if you must use plastic, choose products with a number 2, 4, or 5 listed on the recycle code on the bottom. If the code is not visible, call the company to determine what number the plastic is.

m.   Avoid nonstick or aluminum cookware. Do not use ceramic dishes unless you are certain they are free of lead.

4.   Improve Your Indoor Air

a.   Get house plants such as bamboo palm, Boston fern, chrysanthemum, dwarf date palm, English ivy, ficus, gerbera daisy, golden pothos, peace lily, philodendron, poinsettia, or spider plant.

b.   Enforce a non-smoking rule in your home and cars.

c.   Make sure to properly ventilate your heating source.

d.   Ensure humidity remains below 50 percent.

e.   Ventilate rooms with products that emit formaldehyde or VOCs, such as newly painted rooms and new carpeting.

f.   Have your home inspected for radon.

g.   To order the Indoor Air Quality Community Leader Kit for Women and Children, call the Helpline (800) 557-2366, or go to **http://www.nsc.org/ehc/indoor/wctoc.htm.**

h.   Integrated Pest Management is an alternative to toxic pesticides. Go to **www.ipm.org** for more information.

5.   **Convert Your Home to a Toxin-Free Haven**
     a.   Search the Cosmetics Database at the Environmental Working Group website (**http://www.cosmeticsdatabase.com**) to select healthier personal care products including shampoo, soap, sunscreen, lotion, and baby care products.
     b.   Go to **http://www.beyondpesticides.org/safetysource/index.htm** to search for an integrative pest management provider near you.
     c.   To order a home test kit (about $23) for arsenic go to: **http://www.healthybuilding.net/arsenic/index.html**
     d.   Replace toxic cleaners with safer alternatives, such as baking soda, lemon juice, borax, and vinegar. The Green Guide offers a list of non-toxic cleaners for a variety of cleaning needs. (**www.thegreenguide.com**)
     e.   Open your windows to air the house out instead of spraying air freshener or lighting scented candles.
     f.   Remember that all your trash, fertilizer, and wastewater go back into the groundwater. Dispose of hazardous substances in a responsible manner.
     g.   Look for "green" lawn products and garden services.
     h.   If you swim or own a hot tub, pick a facility or service that uses non-chlorine based disinfectants.
     i.   Plant a tree in the yard and get house plants for inside. According to the Weather Channel's Evening Edition (2/16/07), one tree can remove a ton of carbon dioxide and is equivalent to 10 room-size air conditioners in cooling a home if strategically placed.
     j.   Keep up-to-date on dangerous product recalls at **http://www.recall.gov/**.
     k.   Purchase chlorine-free paper products for writing as well as for coffee filters, paper towels, napkins, tissues, and toilet paper.

6. **Shape up Your Child's School**
    a.   Order the Tools for Schools Action Kit to ensure safer pest control at (800) 438-4318.
    b.   The California School Gardens Networks offers a publication to help you plan, develop, and implement a school garden in your district. More information is available at **http://www.csgn.org/publications.php**. Check out **www.kidsgardening.com** for additional resources. Grants are also available there.
    c.   If you are interested in having The Physician's Committee for Responsible Medicine School Lunch Team work with your school district, go to **http://www.healthyschoollunches.org**.

7. **Have a Healthy Pregnancy**
    a.   Remember that many toxic chemicals are passed through the placenta to a very vulnerable fetus. Follow all of the above recommendations.
    b.   Obtain regular prenatal check-ups.
    c.   Avoid over-the-counter (OTC) medications unless approved by your doctor and be absolutely certain that the benefits of both OTC and prescribed medications outweigh their potential risks. Be especially wary of newer drugs whose problems may not have yet surfaced. Herbal remedies or supplements may not be safe during pregnancy either, so check with a qualified practitioner before using.
    d.   Avoid coloring your hair or going to the hair or nail salon.
    e.   Avoid the dry cleaners and dry cleaned clothing. (If you must wear dry cleaned clothing, remove the plastic and air them out first.)
    f.   Try to avoid all toxic fumes. Have someone else pump your gas, do not refinish furniture or paint the baby's room, don't run the car while it is in the garage, and stay away from home renovation projects. If you find it impossible to avoid

these tasks, wear a mask and be sure the workspace is well-ventilated.

g.   Follow the fish consumption guidelines in your area. Avoid all fish presumed to have a high mercury level.

h.   Eliminate artificial sweeteners.

i.   Do not have silver dental fillings (amalgams) placed or removed while pregnant.

j.   Be sure you are not exposed to any reproductive toxins at work. Request the Hazardous Information Fact Sheets for any chemicals you may be exposed to. (Employers are required by law to provide these to you.)

k.   Visit **www.healthychild.org**

l.   Before registering for your baby shower, check out **www.newbornfree.com** for a selection of safer baby bottles. They offer bisphenol A free plastic bottles as well as glass bottles, training cups, and other products. Evenflo makes glass bottles with silicon nipples.

m.   If you can afford to splurge, consider organic cotton bedding for your newborn. Or add this to your registry.

n.   A gift basket with a copy of this book accompanied by organic baby products makes a great gift for your expectant friends.

o.   When you are finished with this book pass it on to an expectant mother or leave it in the waiting area of your doctor's office.

8.   **Find a Doctor Knowledgeable About Toxins**

a.   Functional medical (FM) providers are treating the root of disease and actually curing chronic diseases! Many of the providers are medical doctors. Several are naturopathic physicians and other clinicians. Just go to **http://www.functionalmedicine.org**, click on search for an FM practitioner, and enter your zipcode.

b.   Clinicians from the American Academy of Environmental Medicine (**www.aaem.com**) are trained to recognize and treat environmental causes of illness.

     c.   Do you have a loved one with autism, Asperger's disease, or somewhere else on the spectrum? Did you know that there are doctors who specialize in the care of these wonderful children? Check out Defeat Autism Now! at **http://www.dan.or**g and find a doctor in your area.

     d.   Check out the International Academy of Oral Medicine and Toxicology to find a doctor/dentist that understands the toxicity of silver fillings at **http://www.iaomt.com**.

9.   **Get Politically Active**

     a.   Stay up-to-date on environmental health concerns. My favorite site is the Environmental working group: **http://www.ewg.org**.

     b.   Visit **http://www.capwiz.com/lcv/dbq/vote_info/**to see how your representatives really feel about the environment.

     c.   Join the Millions Against Monsanto campaign at **http://www.organicconsumers.org/monlink.cfm**.

     d.   Ask your state's legislators what they are doing to protect you and your family. Band together with other concerned citizens and demand protective measures; you may be surprised at what you can achieve. California's many successes in protecting its citizens from toxic harm can surely be replicated in other states.

     e.   Other useful websites include: **www.consumersunion.org, www.whistleblower.com, www.publicintegrity.org, www.corporatepredators.org**.

10.   **Become an "Everyday Activist"**

     a.   Organize a reverse boycott by offering an incentive to the first company in your neighborhood to do something green. For example, the first fast food restaurant to completely eliminate the use of PS foam or plastic to-go containers is saluted in the local paper so that customers will be more likely to patronize that business than its competitors.

b.   Ask your favorite restaurant to offer smaller portion sizes for a slightly reduced price and donate the savings to local food pantries. This omits the need for wasteful, toxic to-go containers.

c.   Place signs in all drive thru windows instructing patrons to turn off their ignition.

d.   Stop idling. Help others to become cognizant of the massive benefit conferred to the planet by simply turning off the car whenever it is not moving.

e.   Start a "Carry Your Cup" campaign in your favorite coffee shop or restaurant. Perhaps the establishments can offer incentives to participants; i.e. every tenth customer to carry her own cup gets her beverage free.

f.   Go to **www.communityhealthaction.org** and learn how to correct a toxic threat in your community. This site offers a toolbox to get you started. This is a great place to begin an investigation about a suspected disease cluster in your hometown.

g.   Check out **www.changemakers.net** if you are considering starting a non-profit organization.

h.   Start a family-matching program where those who are well-to-do purchase healthy food for a less-fortunate family in the community.

i.   Start a community or school edible garden.

j.   Gather your friends and start an "Everyday Activist Book Club." Choose books that keep you informed and empowered to make the world a happier, healthy, more harmonious place for all!

k.   Share your knowledge. Tell everyone you meet how to protect themselves and their families. Lend them this book or send them to

www.holler4health.com for helpful links to begin an action plan of their own.

1.   Visit the Institute for Responsible Technology website at **http://www.responsibletechnology.org** and join the campaign for GM-free schools and communities. While you are there, download a sample letter to take to your favorite restaurants.

*R*ecommended Reading

The UltraSimple Diet by Dr Mark Hyman

I highly recommend this seven-day nourishing detoxification diet because it is simply not possible to avoid all toxins. This is an easy way to shed a few pounds, feel revitalized, and identify foods your body does not respond well to. It may even help you avoid hefty doctor's bills down the road. After completing this short program, you may wish to learn more by reading Dr. Hyman's other excellent books: *Ultrametabolism* and *Ultraprevention.*

The Fat Resistance Diet by Dr. Leo Galland

Discover why diets often fail: The hormone leptin may be the missing link in your weight loss efforts. I am also a big fan of Dr. Galland's *Superimmunity for Kids* and *Four Pillars of Healing.*

The Flavor-Full Diet by David Katz

Learn the science behind food cravings so that you can be prepared to beat them. This book, which is essentially the soft cover version of *The Flavor Point Diet,* provides family-friendly recipes to get you started.

It's All in Your Head by Dr Hal Huggins

Hal Huggins explains how the safe removal of dental fillings can reverse a variety of medical complaints. If you have a mouth full of silver fillings, consider reading this.

The Secret History of the War on Cancer by Devra Davis and *Cancer-Gate: How to Win the Losing Cancer War* by Samuel Epstein

These are real eye-openers about the politics behind the "War on Cancer." Cancer can be prevented and these books reveal why we have yet to accomplish this.

When Smoke Ran Like Water by Devra Davis and *Our Stolen Future: Are We Threatening Our Fertility, Intelligence, and*

Survival? by Theo Colburn, Dianne Dumanoski, and John Peterson Myers

These are two of the books that got me started on the quest to find answers about environmental toxins and health. It was difficult to put either of these books down.

The Newman's Own Organics Guide to a Good Life by Nell Newman

This is a wonderful resource for simple, yet profound, changes that will help save the planet. I think I highlighted the whole book!

What Your Doctor May Not Tell You About Children's Vaccinations by Stephanie Cave M.D. and *Evidence of Harm* by David Kirby

These are two excellent resources that provide information about childhood vaccinations.

The Omnivore's Dilemma: A Natural History of Four Meals and *In Defense of Food: An Eater's Manifesto* by Michael Pollan and *Animal, Vegetable, Miracle: A Year of Food Life* by Barbara Kingsolver, Camille Kingsolver, and Steven Hopp

If you are not yet convinced of the need to eat organic, unprocessed, and locally produced food, these are excellent books to get you motivated.

The Fluoride Deception by Christopher Bryson

This is an excellent resource about the dangers of fluoridated water.

Chapter Notes

Section 1
Chapter 1
1 Landrigan, Philip J, and Carlson, Joy E. "Environmental Policy and Children's Health", The Future of Children. Critical Issues For Children and Youths, Vol 5. No 2. Summer/Fall 1995.
2 Environmental Working Group. "Body Burden: The Pollution of Newborns." July 14, 2005
3 Cassidy Allison and Fidis Alex. Toxic Pollution and Health: An Analysis of Toxic Chemicals Released in Communities Across the United States.Environment California Research and Policy Center. 3/22/2007.
4 National Environmental Trust. Cabinet Confidential: Toxic Products in the Home. Washington DC, July, 2004. Retrieved from http://www.net.org/health/cabcon_report.vtml. Accessed on 5/16/07.

Chapter 2
1 Institute of Functional Medicine website. Retrieved from www.functionalmedicine.org. Accessed on 5/15/07.

Chapter 3
1 Davis, Devra. "When Smoke Ran Like Water: Tales of Environmental Deception and the Battle Against Pollution." Basic Books. 2002.
2 Davis, page 90
3 Davis, page 41-54
4 Davis, page 96
5 US Centers for Disease Control and Prevention. Third National Report on Human Exposure to Environmental Chemicals. 2005.

Chapter 4
1 Epstein Samuel, Gross Liza. "The High Stakes of Cancer Prevention", Tikkun Magazine, Nov/Dec 2000. Retrieved from www.tikkun.org. Accessed on 2/22/07.
2 Retrieved from www.charitynavigator.org. Accessed on 2/22/07.
3 Davis, Devra. When Smoke Ran Like Water. Page 197.
4 Cauchon, D. FDA Advisors Tied to Industry: Approval Process Riddled with Conflicts of Interest. USA TODAY, Sept. 25, 2000
5 Sardi, Bill. Just How Many Americans Did Vioxx Kill? April 21,2006. Retrieved from http://www.lewrockwell.com/sardi/sardi53.html. Accessed on 10/4/07.
6 Public Citizen. Petition to the FDA to issue strong warnings about the potential for certain cholesterol-lowering drugs to cause potentially life-threatening muscle damage. (HRG Publication #1588). August 20, 2001. Retrieved from http://www.citizen.org/publications/release.cfm?ID=7051. Accessed on 10/4/07
7 The National Institutes of Health. Women's Health Initiative.

Section 2
1 Center for Disease Control and Prevention. Chronic Disease Overview.
11/18/2005
Retrieved from National Center for Chronic Disease Prevention and Health
Promotion http://www.cdc.gov/nccdphp/overview.htm. Accessed on
3/31/06.
2 JAMA 2003;290:1884-1890.
3 Merck Institute of Aging and Health. "The State of Aging and Health in
America 2004". Washington DC. 2004.

Chapter 6
1 Meggs William J. Neurogenic Inflammation and Sensitivity to
Environmental Chemicals. Environmental Health Perspectives.Volume
101, Number 3, August 1993. Retrieved from
http://www.ehponline.org/members/1993/101-3/meggs-full.html.
Accessed on 5/18/07.
2 Life Extension website. www.lef.org. accessed on 5/18/07.
3 Duncan BB, Schmidt MI, Pankow JI, et al. Low-grade systemic
inflammation and the development of type 2 diabetes. The Atherosclerosis
Risk in Communities study. Diabetes 2003;52:1799-1805.
4 Licinio J, Wong ML. The role of inflammatory mediators in the biology of
major depression: central nervous system cytokines modulate the
biological substrate of depressive symptoms, regulate stress-responsive
systems, and contribute to neurotoxicity and neuroprotection. Mol
Psychiatry 1999 Jul; 4(4):317-27
5 Harris RE, Chlebowski RT, Jackson RD, et al. Breast cancer and
nonsteroidal anti-inflammatory drugs: prospective results from the
Women's Health Initiative. Cancer Res. 2003;63:6096-6101.
6 Knopper, Melissa. Auto exposure: Do immune system diseases have an
environmental cause? The Environmental Magazine. May-June, 2005.
7 CDC. Prevalence of disability and associated health conditions—United
States, 1991–1992. MMWR 1994;43(40): 730–1, 737–9.
8 Harr, Jonathan. A Civil Action. p 246.
9 National Institutes of Health.
10 Ross, Peter. The Role of Immunotoxic Environmental Contaminants in
Facilitating the Emergence of Infectious Diseases in Marine Mammals.
Human and Ecological Risk Assessment, Volume 8, Issue 2 April 2002 ,
pages 277 – 292.
11 Davis, Devra. When Smoke Ran Like Water.
12 Reilly, Michael. "Pollutant damages child immunity. (This week:
International news and exclusives)." New Scientist 191.2566 (August 26,
2006): 12(1). Expanded Academic ASAP. Thomson Gale. Remote Access. 9
Mar. 2007.
12 Hyman, Mark. Ultrametabolism. Scribner, an Imprint of Simon &
Schuster, Inc., N.Y. 2006.
13 Mercury-induced autoimmunity in mice. Nielsen J B and Hultman P.
Environ Health Perspect. 2002 October; 110(Suppl 5): 877–881.
14 Colburn, Theo, Dianne Dumanoski, and John Peterson Myers and John
Peterson Myers Our Stolen Future. Dutton, Peguin Books. 1996.

Chapter 7
1 Colburn, Theo. Our Stolen Future. Page 39.
2 Bauer, Rosemary, Colburn Theo, Palanza Paola, Parmigiani Stefano, vom Saal Frederick. Endocrine Disruptors. Environmental Health Perspectives. Volume 110 (3). June 2002.
3 World Health Organization. Global Assessment of the State-of-the-Science of Endocrine Disruptors. 2002.
4 Sugiura-Ogasawara M, Ozaki Y, Sonta S, Makino T, Suzumori K. Exposure to bisphenol A is associated with recurrent miscarriage. Human Reproduction 2005; 20(8):2325-9
5 Stahlhut Richard W, Wijngaarden Edwin van, Dye Timothy D, Cook Stephen, and Swan Shanna H. Concentrations of Urinary Phthalate Metabolites Are Associated with Increased Waist Circumference and Insulin Resistance in Adult U.S. Males. Environmental Health Perspectives Volume 115, Number 6, June 2007. Retrieved from http://www.ehponline.org/docs/2007/9882/abstract.html. Accessed on June 6, 2007.
6 Stemp-Morlock Graeme. Exploring Developmental Origins of Obesity. Environmental Health Perspectives Volume 115, Number 5, May 2007. Retrieved from http://www.ehponline.org/docs/2007/115-5/forum.html#expl. Accessed on 6/1/07.
7 Mills, Dixie. Endocrine Disruptors: Tipping the Hormonal Scales. 2/9/07. Retrieved from http://www.womentowomen.com/detoxification/endocrinedisruptors.asp. Accessed on 5/10/07.

Chapter 8
1 Grandjean and Landrigan PJ. Developmental neurotoxicity of industrial chemicals. The Lancet. 368.9553 (12). Dec 16, 2006. p2167.
2 Hock C, Drasch G, Golombowski S, Muller-Spahn F, Willershausen-Zonnchen B, Schwarz P, Hock U, Growdon J.H, Nitsch R.M. "Increased Blood Mercury Levels in Patients with Alzheimer's Disease" Journal of Neural Transmission, 105: (1998).
3 Wastenssona G, Hagberga S, Anderssona E, Johnelsb B, Barregarda L. Parkinson's disease in diphenyl-exposed workers-A causal association? Volume 12, Issue 1, Pages 29-34 January 2006.
4 Cassidy Allison and Fidis Alex. Toxic Pollution and Health: An Analysis of Toxic Chemicals Released in Communities Across the United States.Environment California Research and Policy Center. 3/22/2007.
5 Orr L. PCBs, fungicide open brain cells to Parkinson's assault.University of Rochester Medical Center. 10 Feb 2005. Retrieved from http://www.urmc.rochester.edu. Accessed on 3/16/07.
6 Wright J Michael and Keller-Bryne Jane. Environmental Determinants of Parkinson's Disease. Archives of Environmental and Occupational Health. 1/1/05. Retrieved from http://www.accessmylibrary.com/coms2/summary_0286-17664594_ITM. Accessed on 5/17/07.

7 Di Monte DA, Lavasani M, Manning-Bog AB. Environmental factors in Parkinson's disease. The Parkinson's Institute, Sunnyvale, CA.
8 Grandjean and Landrigan PJ. Developmental neurotoxicity of industrial chemicals. The Lancet. 368.9553 (12). Dec 16, 2006. p2167.
9 National Research Council. Biological markers in immunotoxicology. Autoimmune diseases. Washington, DC:National Academy Press, 1992.
10 Ascherio A, Chen H, Weisskopf MG, O'Reilly E, McCullough ML, Calle EE, Schwarzschild MA, Thun MJ. Pesticide exposure and risk for Parkinson's disease. Ann Neurol. 2006 Aug; 60(2):197-203.
11 Wikipedia.
12 Wright J Michael and Keller-Bryne Jane. Environmental Determinants of Parkinson's Disease. Archives of Environmental and Occupational Health. 1/1/05. Retrieved from http://www.accessmylibrary.com/coms2/summary_0286-17664594_ITM. Accessed on 5/17/07.
13 Cassidy Allison and Fidis Alex. Toxic Pollution and Health: An Analysis of Toxic Chemicals Released in Communities Across the United States.Environment California Research and Policy Center. 3/22/2007.
14 Skegg DCG. Multiple sclerosis: nature or nurture? (New evidence reaffirms the importance of environmental factors) (editorial). British Medical Journal 302.6771. Feb 2, 1991. p247(2).
15 Skegg DCG. Multiple sclerosis: nature or nurture? (New evidence reaffirms the importance of environmental factors) (editorial). British Medical Journal 302.6771. Feb 2, 1991. p247(2).
16 Mercury and MS. Swed J Biol Med. January 1989.
17 B12 and MS. J Appl Nutri, 1973; 25: 16-40.
 Lancet, 26 May, 1990.
18 B12 and MS. Int Med, 1994; 33: 82-6.
19 Pipher Mary. Reviving Ophelia: Saving the Selves of Adolescent Girls. Ballantine Books. 1995.
p 94.
20 National Institute of Mental Health.1998.
21 Slotkin Theodore A, Tate Charlotte A, Ryde Ian T, Levin Edward D,and Seidler Frederic J. Organophosphate Insecticides Target the Serotonergic System in Developing Rat Brain Regions: Disparate Effects of Diazinon and Parathion at Doses Spanning the Threshold for Cholinesterase Inhibition. Environmental Health Perspectives Volume 114, Number 10, October 2006. Retrieved from http://www.ehponline.org/members/2006/9337/9337.html. Accessed on 6/5/07.
22 Grum Darja Kobal, Kobal Alfred B, Arneric Niko, Horvat Milena, Zenko Bernard, Dzeroski Saso and Osredkar Josko. Personality Traits in Miners with Past Occupational Elemental Mercury Exposure. Environmental Health Perspectives Volume 114, Number 2, February 2006. Retrieved from http://www.ehponline.org/members/2006/7863/7863.html. Accessed on 6/5/07.
23 World Health Organization. 1976, 1991, 2003.
24 Spivey A. Increased suicide rate with possible link to nearby industry chemicals in second N.C. community, USA. Nov 10 2005.

Chapter Notes

25 Boffetta et al. 1998.

26 National Center for Injury Prevention and Control. Fact Book. Atlanta, Ga. 2006.

27 Tuormaa, Tuula. The adverse effects of food additives on health: With a special emphasis on childhood hyperactivity. Journal of Orthomolecular Medicine. 9(4) 225-243. 1994.

28 Soffritti M, Belpoggi F, Tibaldi E, Esposti DD, and Lauriola M. Life-Span Exposure to Low Doses of Aspartame Beginning during Prenatal Life Increases Cancer Effects in Rats. Environ Health Perspect 115:1293–1297 (2007). Online 13 June 2007.

29 Center for Science in the Public Interest. Retrieved from http://www.cspinet.org/reports/chemcuisine.htm. Accessed on 7/7/07

30 Center for Science in the Public Interest. Retrieved from http://www.cspinet.org/reports/chemcuisine.htm. Accessed on 7/7/07

31 Nissen, Steven. ADHD Drugs and Cardiovascular Risk. The New England Journal of Medicine. 354;14. April 6, 2006. 1445-48

32 Nissen, Steven. ADHD Drugs and Cardiovascular Risk. The New England Journal of Medicine. 354;14. April 6, 2006. 1445-48

33 Center for Science in the Public Interest. Retrieved from http://www.cspinet.org/reports/chemcuisine.htm. Accessed on 7/7/07

34 Starobrat-Hermelin B. [The effect of deficiency of selected bioclements on hyperactivity in children with certain specified mental disorders]. Ann Acad Med Stetin 1998; 44:297-314

Chapter 9

1 Schettler T, Stein J, Reich F, and Valenti M for Greater Boston Physicians for Social Responsibility. In Harm's Way: Toxic Threats to Child Development. Cambridge, MA May 2000. retrieved from http://www.igc.org/psr/. Accessed on January 28, 2006.

2 Schettler T, Stein J, Reich F, and Valenti M for Greater Boston Physicians for Social Responsibility. In Harm's Way: Toxic Threats to Child Development. Cambridge, MA May 2000. retrieved from http://www.igc.org/psr/. Accessed on January 28, 2006.

3 Grandjean and Landrigan PJ. Developmental neurotoxicity of industrial chemicals. The Lancet. 368.9553 (12). Dec 16, 2006. p2167.

4 Grandjean and Landrigan PJ. Developmental neurotoxicity of industrial chemicals. The Lancet. 368.9553 (12). Dec 16, 2006. p2167.

5 Learning Disabilities Association of America (LDA), the National Education Association (NEA), and the Arc of the United States. Mercury and Learning Disabilities: A Parent's Guide. March 14, 2005. Retrieved from http://cta.policy.net/proactive/newsroom/release.vtml?id=25831. Accessed on 4/17/07.

6 K. Crump, T. Kjellstrom, A. Shipp, A. Silvers, and A. Stewart, "Influence of Prenatal Mercury Exposure upon Scholastic and Psychological Test Performance: Benchmark Analysis of a New Zealand Cohort," Risk Analysis 18, no. 6(1998): 701-13.

P. Grandjean et al., "Cognitive Deficit in Seven-Year-Old Children with Prenatal Exposure to MeHg," Neurotoxicology and Teratology 19, no. 6 (1997):417-28.

7 Harada H. Congenital Minamata disease: intrauterine methylmercury poisoning. Teratology 18:285-288.
Amin-Zaki L, Ehassani S, Majeed MA, Clarkson T, Doherty R, Greenwood M, Giovanoli-Jakubezak T. 1976. Perinatal methylmercury poisoning in Iraq. Am J Dis Child 130:1070-1076.
8 Rice DC. 1998. Developmental lead exposure: neurobehavioral consequences. In: Handbook of Developmental Neurotoxicology (Slikker W, Chang LW, eds). San Diego, CA:Academic Press.
Needleman HL, Reiss JA, Tobin MJ, Biesecher G, Greenhouse J. 1996. Bone lead levels and delinquent behavior. JAMA 275:363-369.
9 Lanphear Bruce P. Dietrich KN, Auinger P, Cox C. Cognitive Deficits Associated with Blood Lead Levels Less than 10 ug/dl in US Children and Adolescents. Public Health Rep. 115:521-529. 2000.
10 Lanphear et al. 2000.
11 Collipp PJ, Chen SY, Maitinsky S. Manganese in infant formulas and learning disability. Ann Nutri Metab 27:488-494.
Pihl RO, Parkes M. 1977. Hair element content in learning disabled children. Science 198:204-206 (1977).
Ericson JE. 1998. Manganese, aggression, and attention-deficit hyperactivity disorder. Neurotoxicology 19(3):468-469.
12 Jacobson JL, Jacobson SW. 1990. Effects of in utero exposure to PCBs and related contaminants on cognitive functioning in young children. J Pediatr 116(1):38-45. Jacobson JL, Jacobson SW. 1996. Intellectual impairment in children exposed to polychlorinated biphenyls in utero. N Engl J Med 335:783-789.
Patandin et al. 1999;
Lonky E, Reihman J, Darvill T. 1996. Neonatal behavioral assessment scale performance in humans influenced by maternal consumption of environmentally contaminated Lake Ontario fish. J Great Lakes Res 22(2):198-212.Stewart et al. 2000,
Rice DC, Hayward S. 1997. Effects of postnatal exposure to a PCB mixture in monkeys on nonspatial discrimination reversal and delayed alternation performance. NeuroToxicology 18(2):479-494. Rice DC. 1999. Behavioral impairment produced by low-level postnatal PCB exposure in monkeys. Environ Res (sect A) 80:S113-121.
13 Grandjean and Landrigan PJ. Developmental neurotoxicity of industrial chemicals. The Lancet. 368.9553 (12). Dec 16, 2006. p2167.

Chapter 10
1 CDC, Eliminate Disparities, 2007
2 Radiation and Public Health Project, Brooklyn, NY. New York Times Article Discusses Rise in Childhood Cancers. Retrieved from http://www.chem-tox.com/cancerchildren/. Accessed March 1, 2006.
3 Gouveia-Vigeant, Tami and Tickner, Joel. Toxic Chemicals and Childhood Cancer : A Review of the Evidence. Lowell Center for Sustainable Production. University of Massachusetts Lowell. 5/2003.
4 Lichtenstein P et al. Environmental and Heritable Factors in the Causation of Cancer. NEJM. 2000.
5 CDC, 20 Leading Causes of Death 2003

6 Mangano JJ. A Rise in the Incidence of Childhood Cancer in the United States. Interantional Journal of Health Services. 1999. 29 (2) 393-408.

7 Gouveia-Vigeant, Tami and Tickner, Joel. 2003

8 Mangano JJ. A Rise in the Incidence of Childhood Cancer in the United States. Interantional Journal of Health Services. 1999. 29 (2) 393-408.

9 Gouveia-Vigeant, Tami and Tickner, Joel. 2003.

10 Harr, Jonathan. A Civil Action.

11 Gouveia-Vigeant, Tami and Tickner, Joel. 2003.

12 Mills PK, Yang R. Regression analysis of pesticide use and breast cancer incidence in California. Latinas. J Environ Health. 68(6):15-22 . 2006.

13 Sarasua, Sara and Savitz, David. Cured and Broiled Meat Consumption in Relation to Childhood Cancer: Denver, Colorado. (United States). Cancer Causes & Control, Vol. 5, No. 2 (Mar., 1994), pp. 141-148

14 Gale, Karin B et al. Backtracking Leukemia to Birth: Identification of Clonotypic Gene Fusion Sequences in Neonatal Blood Spots. Proceedings of the National Academy of Sciences of the United States of America, Volume 94, Issue 25, pp. 13950-13954. 12/1997.

15 Sarasua, Sara and Savitz, David. Cured and Broiled Meat Consumption in Relation to Childhood Cancer: Denver, Colorado. (United States). Cancer Causes & Control, Vol. 5, No. 2 (Mar., 1994), pp. 141-148

16 CDC, 2003

17 The American Cancer Society's Surveillance Research, 2006

18 Environmental and Occupational Causes of Cancer: A Review of Recent Scientific Literature. Lowell Center for Sustainable Production. September 2005.

19 Environmental and Occupational Causes of Cancer.

20 Environmental and Occupational Causes of Cancer.

21 Environmental and Occupational Causes of Cancer.

22 Brody JG, Rudel RA. 2003. Environmental Pollutants and Breast Cancer. Environmental Health Perspectives. 111:1007-19.

23 Boyce, JD for Sprecher Institute for Comparative Cancer Resesarch. Ionizing Radiation and Breast Cancer Risk. Fact Sheet #52. Program on Breast Cancer and Environmental Risk Factors. January 2005.

24 Environmental and Occupational Causes of Cancer.

25 Environmental and Occupational Causes of Cancer.

26 Environmental and Occupational Causes of Cancer.

27 Environmental and Occupational Causes of Cancer.

28 Environmental and Occupational Causes of Cancer.

29 Environmental and Occupational Causes of Cancer.

30 Davis, Devra. When Smoke Ran Like Water. p 100.

31 Arden Pope et al. "Lung Cancer, Cardiopulmonary Mortality, and Long-term Exposure to Fine Particulate Air Pollution."JAMA march 2002.

32 Davis Devra. When Smoke Ran Like Water. p 100.

33 Environmental and Occupational Causes of Cancer.

34 Epstein. p 4.

35 Landrigan, 2002, Environmental pollutants and disease in American Children

36 Landrigan, 2002, Environmental pollutants and disease in American Children

Chapter 11

1 Tuormaa, Tuula. The adverse effects of food additives on health: With a special emphasis on childhood hyperactivity. Journal of Orthomolecular Medicine. 9(4) 225-243. 1994.
2 Center for Science in the Public Interest. Retrieved from http://www.cspinet.org/reports/chemcuisine.htm. Accessed on 7/7/07.
3 Center for Science in the Public Interest. Retrieved from http://www.cspinet.org/reports/chemcuisine.htm. Accessed on 7/7/07.
4 Sarasua, Sara and Savitz, David. Cured and Broiled Meat Consumption in Relation to Childhood Cancer: Denver, Colorado. (United States). Cancer Causes & Control, Vol. 5, No. 2 (Mar., 1994), pp. 141-148
5 Center for Science in the Public Interest. Retrieved from http://www.cspinet.org/reports/chemcuisine.htm. Accessed on 7/7/07.
6 Center for Science in the Public Interest. Retrieved from http://www.cspinet.org/reports/chemcuisine.htm. Accessed on 7/7/07.
7 Soffritti M, Belpoggi F, Tibaldi E, Esposti DD, and Lauriola M. Life-Span Exposure to Low Doses of Aspartame Beginning during Prenatal Life Increases Cancer Effects in Rats. Environ Health Perspect 115:1293–1297 (2007). Online 13 June 2007.
8 Soffritti M, Belpoggi F, Tibaldi E, Esposti DD, and Lauriola M. Life-Span Exposure to Low Doses of Aspartame Beginning during Prenatal Life Increases Cancer Effects in Rats. Environ Health Perspect 115:1293–1297 (2007). Online 13 June 2007.
9 Soffritti M, Belpoggi F, Tibaldi E, Esposti DD, and Lauriola M. Life-Span Exposure to Low Doses of Aspartame Beginning during Prenatal Life Increases Cancer Effects in Rats. Environ Health Perspect 115:1293–1297 (2007). Online 13 June 2007.
10 Center for Science in the Public Interest. Retrieved from http://www.cspinet.org/reports/chemcuisine.htm. Accessed on 7/7/07.
11 FAQs about Food Irradiation: Registered Dietitian, Karen Graham answers some questions. Retrieved from http://www.citizen.org/cmep/foodsafety/international/canada/articles.cfm?ID=9532
12 Parnes, Robin Brett, William C. Idell, Audrey L. Anastasia Kanik, and Alice H. Lichtenstein. Food irradiation: an overlooked opportunity for food safety and preservation. Nutrition Today. 38.5 (Sept-Oct 2003):174(12). Expanded Academic ASAP. Gale. Remote Access. 15 Aug. 2007
13 FAQs about Food Irradiation: Registered Dietitian, Karen Graham answers some questions. Retrieved from http://www.citizen.org/cmep/foodsafety/international/canada/articles.cfm?ID=9532
14 Parnes, Robin Brett, William C. Idell, Audrey L. Anastasia Kanik, and Alice H. Lichtenstein. Food irradiation: an overlooked opportunity for food safety and preservation. Nutrition Today. 38.5 (Sept-Oct 2003):174(12). Expanded Academic ASAP. Gale. Remote Access. 15 Aug. 2007

15 Parnes, Robin Brett, William C. Idell, Audrey L. Anastasia Kanik, and Alice H. Lichtenstein. Food irradiation: an overlooked opportunity for food safety and preservation. Nutrition Today. 38.5 (Sept-Oct 2003):174(12). Expanded Academic ASAP. Gale. Remote Access. 15 Aug. 2007

16 Dougherty Charlotte P, Holtz Sarah Hendricks Reinert Joseph C, Panyacosit Lily, Axelrad Daniel A and Woodruff Tracey J. Dietary Exposure to Food Contaminants across the United States. Environmental Research Section A. 84, 170-185. 2000.

17 Gouveia-Vigeant, Tami and Tickner, Joel. Toxic Chemicals and Childhood Cancer : A Review of the Evidence. Lowell Center for Sustainable Production. University of Massachusetts Lowell. 5/2003.

18 Chan, June M., et. al., "Plasma Insulin-Like Growth Factor-1 [IGF-1] and Prostate Cancer Risk: A Prospective Study," Science, vol. 279, January 23, 1998, pp. 563-566

19 Hankinson, S. E., et. al., "Circulating concentrations of insulin-like growth factor 1 and risk of breast cancer," Lancet, vol. 351, no. 9113, 1998, pp. 1393-1396

20 Mepham T. B., et al., "Safety of milk from cows treated with bovine somatotropin," Lancet, Vol. 344, November 19, 1994, pp. 1445-1446

21 Smith, J. Whistleblowers, threats, and bribes: a short history of genetically engineered bovine growth hormone. Genewatch. 2005 May-Jun;18(3):6-9, 16

22 Roseboro, Ken. Monsanto Pressures FDA To Keep Consumers In The Dark. Non GMO News. August 6, 2007. Retrieved from http://www.enn.com/top_stories/article/21395. Accesed on 8/17/07.

23 www.organicconsumers.org

24 www.ewg.org

25 Environmental Working Group. "Body Burden: The Pollution of Newborns." July 14, 2005

26 http://www.pristineplanet.com/newsletter/2006/05.asp

27http://en.wikipedia.org/wiki/Bradford_sweets_poisoning

Chapter 12

1 www.soilassociation.org

2 Pew Initiative on Food and Biotechnology. Feeding the World: A Look at Biotechnology and World Hunger. Washington DC. March, 2004.

3 Pew Initiative on Food and Biotechnology. Feeding the World: A Look at Biotechnology and World Hunger. Washington DC. March, 2004.

4 Pew Initiative on Food and Biotechnology. Feeding the World: A Look at Biotechnology and World Hunger. Washington DC. March, 2004.

5 Friends of the Earth website. www.foe.org

6 Genetically Modified Crops and Illness Linked. Manila Bulletin. 04-Mar-2004. Retrieved from http://www.seedquest.com/News/releases/2004/march/8017.htm. Accessed on 7/24/07.

7 Sarmiento Romer S. 'BT' Toxin Found in B'Laans" Blood. Philippines Today. March 5, 2004. Retrieved from http://www.seedquest.com/News/releases/2004/march/8017.htm. Accessed on 7/24/07.

8 B'Laan Farmer Blames GMO Corn for Coughs, Nausea, Even Rashes. Manila Bulletin. 05-Mar-2004. Retrieved from http://www.seedquest.com/News/releases/2004/march/8017.htm. Accessed on 7/24/07.
9 Séralini, G-E, Cellier, D. & Spiroux de Vendomois, J. 2007. New analysis of a rat feeding study with a genetically modified maize reveals signs of hepatorenal toxicity. Published in: "Archives of Environmental Contamination and Toxicology". Greenpeace website.
10 www.soilassociation.org
11 Freese, Bill for Friends of the Earth. "Manufacturing Drugs and Chemicals in Crops: Biopharming poses New Threats to Consumers, Farmers, Food Companies and the Environment. Genetically Engineered Food Alert. July, 2002. Retrieved from www.foe.org/biopharm. Accessed on 7/23/07.
12 Lancet. May 29, 1999.
13 Institute for Responsible Technology Website: http://www.responsibletechnology.org

Chapter 13
1 Environmental Working Group. In The Drink. 1995
2 Environmental Working Group. A National Assessment of Tap Water Quality. December 20, 2005
3 Environmental Working Group. A National Assessment of Tap Water Quality. December 20, 2005
4 Environmental Working Group. A National Assessment of Tap Water Quality. December 20, 2005
5 National Resources Defense Council. Tap Water Quality and Safety. June 11, 2003. Retrieved from http://www.nrdc.org/water/drinking/qtap.asp. Accessed May 30, 2006.
6 Environmental Working Group. A National Assessment of Tap Water Quality. December 20, 2005
7 Sharp, Renee and Walker, Bill. Rocket Science: Perchlorate and the Toxic Legacy of the Cold War. Environmental Working Group. July, 2001.
8 Sharp, Renee and Walker, Bill. Rocket Science: Perchlorate and the Toxic Legacy of the Cold War. Environmental Working Group. July, 2001.
9 Sharp, Renee and Walker, Bill. Rocket Science: Perchlorate and the Toxic Legacy of the Cold War. Environmental Working Group. July, 2001.
10 Broome, Gerry. Congress probes tainted water at N.C. base. Associated Press. Washington. June 12, 2007
Retrieved from http://www.msnbc.msn.com/id/19189878/Accessed on 6/14/07.
11 Gouveia-Vigeant, Tami and Tickner, Joel. Toxic Chemicals and Childhood Cancer : A Review of the Evidence. Lowell Center for Sustainable Production. University of Massachusetts Lowell. 5/2003.
12 Zahm SH, Ward MH., Pesticides and childhood cancer, in Environ Health, in Perspect.1998 Jun;106 Suppl 3:893-908.
13 J.R. Self and R.M. Waskom. Nitrates in Drinking Water. July 1995. Updated Wednesday, July 12, 2006 Colorado State University Cooperative Extension. no. 0.517. Retrieved from

Chapter Notes

http://www.ext.colostate.edu/PUBS/crops/00517.html. Accessed on 6/14/07.
14 J.R. Self and R.M. Waskom. Nitrates in Drinking Water. July 1995. Updated Wednesday, July 12, 2006 Colorado State University Cooperative Extension. no. 0.517. Retrieved from http://www.ext.colostate.edu/PUBS/crops/00517.html. Accessed on 6/14/07.
15 J.R. Self and R.M. Waskom. Nitrates in Drinking Water. July 1995. Updated Wednesday, July 12, 2006 Colorado State University Cooperative Extension. no. 0.517. Retrieved from http://www.ext.colostate.edu/PUBS/crops/00517.html. Accessed on 6/14/07.
16 J.R. Self and R.M. Waskom. Nitrates in Drinking Water. July 1995. Updated Wednesday, July 12, 2006 Colorado State University Cooperative Extension. no. 0.517. Retrieved from http://www.ext.colostate.edu/PUBS/crops/00517.html. Accessed on 6/14/07.
17 J.R. Self and R.M. Waskom. Nitrates in Drinking Water. July 1995. Updated Wednesday, July 12, 2006 Colorado State University Cooperative Extension. no. 0.517. Retrieved from http://www.ext.colostate.edu/PUBS/crops/00517.html. Accessed on 6/14/07.
18 Wikipedia
19 Environmental Working Group. MTBE Groundwater Contamination. http://www.ewg.org/node/21314.
20 Environmental Working Group. MTBE Groundwater Contamination. http://www.ewg.org/node/21314.
21 Field RW, Steck DJ, Smith BJ, Brus CP, Neuberger JS, Fisher EF, Platz CE, Robinson RA, Woolson RF, Lynch CF. Residential Radon Gas Exposure and Lung Cancer: The Iowa Radon Lung Cancer Study. American Journal of Epidemiology. 151(11):1091-1102. 2000.
22 http://en.wikipedia.org/wiki/Arsenic
23 http://en.wikipedia.org/wiki/Arsenicosis
24 http://en.wikipedia.org/wiki/Arsenic
25 http://www.safe-drinking-water.org
26 Agency for Toxic Substances and Disease Registry. Case Studies in Environmental Medicine (CSEM). Retrieved from http://www.atsdr.cdc.gov/HEC/CSEM/arsenic/cover.html#alert. Accessed on 8/11/07.
27 http://www.safe-drinking water.org/as_health.html
28 San-Xiang Wang, Zheng-Hui Wang, Xiao-Tian Cheng, Jun Li, Zhi-Ping Sang, Xiang-Dong Zhang, Ling-Ling Han, Xiao-Yan Qiao, Zhao-Ming Wu, and Zhi-Quan Wang. Arsenic and Fluoride Exposure in Drinking Water: Children's IQ and Growth in Shanyin County, Shanxi Province, China. Environmental Health Perspectives Volume 115, Number 4, April 2007.
29 Environmental Working Group. Chrome-Plated Fraud: How PG&E's Scientists-For-Hire Reversed Findings of Cancer Study. December 23, 2005. Retrieved from http://www.ewg.org/reports/chromium. Acessed on 8/11/07.

219

30 National Toxicology Program. Hexavalent Chromium in Drinking Water Causes Cancer in Lab Animals. NIH News. 5/16/07. Retrieved from http://www.nih.gov/news/pr/may2007/niehs-16.htm. Accessed on 8/11/07.
31 Environmental Working Group. Chrome-Plated Fraud: How PG&E's Scientists-For-Hire Reversed Findings of Cancer Study. December 23, 2005. Retrieved from http://www.ewg.org/reports/chromium. Acessed on 8/11/07.
32 http://www.cyber-nook.com/water/contam.html
33 Schettler T, Stien J, Reich F, Valenti M for Greater Boston Physicians for Social Responsibility. In Harm's Way: Toxic Threats to Child Development. Cambridge, MA. May 2000. Retrieved from http://www.igc.org/psr/. Accessed on January 28, 2006.
34 Schettler T, Stien J, Reich F, Valenti M for Greater Boston Physicians for Social Responsibility. In Harm's Way: Toxic Threats to Child Development. Cambridge, MA. May 2000. Retrieved from http://www.igc.org/psr/. Accessed on January 28, 2006.
35 Water Quality Inventory, EPA 2000
36 Faust and Aly. Chemistry of Water Treatment. Ann Arbor Press. Chelsea, MI. 1998.
37 Olson, Erik D. for National Resources Defense Council. Bottled Water: Pure Drink or Pure Hype? February 1999. Retrieved from http://www.nrdc.org/water/drinking/bw/bwinx.asp. Accessed on 8/12/07.
38 Olson, Erik D.
39 Olson, Erik D.
40 WaterWeek Authors. Mayors to examine bottled water impacts. 07/02/2007. Retrieved from http://www.awwa.org/Communications/news/. Accessed on 7/11/07.
41 Schettler T, Stien J, Reich F, Valenti M for Greater Boston Physicians for Social Responsibility. In Harm's Way: Toxic Threats to Child Development. Cambridge, MA. May 2000. Retrieved from http://www.igc.org/psr/. Accessed on January 28, 2006.

Chapter 14
1 Centers for Disease Control and Prevention. Populations Receiving Optimally Fluoridated Public Drinking Water- United States, 2000. Morbidity and Mortality Weekly Report. February 22, 2002 / 51(07);144-7.
2 Stride S. Honolulu Bans Water Fluoridation. Citizens for Safe Drinking Water. March 4, 2004. Retrieved from http://www.Keepers-of-the-Well.org. Accessed on 7/21/07.
3 Peterson Poul Erik for the World Health Organization. The World Oral Health Report 2003: Continuous Improvement of Oral Health in the 21st Century- The approach of the WHO Global Oral Health Programme. 2003.
4 www.flouridation.com contains numerous references

5 Maupomé G, Clark DC, Levy SM, Berkowitz J. Patterns of dental caries following the cessation of water fluoridation. Community Dent Oral Epidemiol 2001 Feb;29(1):37-47. Faculty of Dentistry, University of British Columbia.

6 Sutton Philip RN, The Greatest Fraud Fluoridation, 1996
7 Centers for Disease Control and Prevention. Surveillance for Dental
Caries, Dental Sealants, Tooth Retention, Edentulism, and Enamel
Fluorosis --- United States, 1988--1994 and 1999—2002. Morbidity and
Mortality Weekly Report. August 26, 2005. 54(03);1-44 (2005). Retrieved
from
http://www.cdc.gov/mmwr/preview/mmwrhtml/ss5403a1.htm#tab23.
Accessed on 7/23/07.
8 Hong L, Levy SM, et al. (2006). Timing of fluoride intake in relation to
development of fluorosis on maxillary central incisors. Community
Dentistry and Oral Epidemiology 34:299-309.
9 Danielson, C., Lyon, J.L., Egger, M., and Goodenough, G.K. Hip fracture
and fluoridation in Utah's elderly population. JAMA 268 746-748 (1992).
Jacobsen, S.J., Goldberg, J., Miles, ,T.P. et al. Regional variation in the
incidence of hip fracture: U.S. white women aged 65 years and older.
JAMA 264 500-502 (1990)
Orcel P, et al. (1990). Stress fractures of the lower limbs in osteoporotic
patients treated with fluoride. Journal of Bone and Mineral Research
5(Suppl 1): S191-4.

10 Spittle B, Psychopharmacology of fluoride: a review, Int Clin
Psychopharmacol, 9:2, 1994 Summer, 79-82

11 Li, X.S., Zhi, J.L., and Gao, R.O. Effect of fluoride exposure on
intelligence in children. Fluoride 28 (1995).
Wang SX, et al. (2007). Water arsenic and fluoride exposure and children's
intelligence quotient and growth in Shanyin County, Shanxi, China.
Environmental Health Perspectives [Epub Jan 9].
Zhao, L.B., Liang, G.H., Zhang, D.N., and Wu, X.R.Effect of high fluoride
water supply on children's intelligence. Fluoride 29 190-192 (1996)
12 Cheng YX, IQ of children in areas of high fluorine content, Chinese
Journal of Control of Endemic Diseases, Supplement 1991.
13 He H, Chen ZS, Liu XM, The effects of fluoride on the human embryo,
Chinese Journal of Control of Epidemic Diseases, 1989, 4, 136-137.
14 Xiong X, et al. (2007). Dose-effect relationship between drinking water
fluoride levels and damage to liver and kidney functions in children.
Environmental Research 103:112-116. (Reviewed in: American Academy of
Pediatrics (AAP) Grand Rounds; 2007; 17:7).
15 Luke, J.A. Effect of fluoride on the physiology of the pineal gland.
Caries Research 28 204 (1994).
16 Bassin EB, Wypij D, Davis RB, Mittleman MA. (2006). Age-specific
Fluoride Exposure in Drinking Water and Osteosarcoma (United States).
Cancer Causes and Control 17: 421-8.
Cohn PD. (1992). A Brief Report On The Association Of Drinking Water
Fluoridation And The Incidence of Osteosarcoma Among Young Males. New
Jersey Department of Health Environ. Health Service: 1- 17.
Tsutsui et al. Chromosome aberrations, sister chromatid exchanges,
unscheduled DNA synthesis and morphological neoplastic transformation
in Syrian hamster embryo cells. Cancer Research 44 938-941 (1984).

221

17 Science and Public Policy. An increase in the number of Down's syndrome babies born to younger mothers in cities following fluoridation. 36-46 (1985).

18 National Research Council. (2006). Fluoride in Drinking Water: A Scientific Review of EPA's Standards. National Academies Press, Washington D.C.

19 National Research Council. 2006.

20 National Research Council. 2006.

21 National Research Council. 2006.

22 National Research Council. 2006.

23 National Research Council. 2006.

24 Connett Michael. The Phosphate Fertilizer Industry: An Environmental Overview.Fluoride Action Network. May 2003. Retrieved from http://www.fluoridealert.org/phosphate/overview.htm. Accessed on 7/22/07.

25 Hanmer Rebecca. Letter to Deputy Assistant Administrator for Water, to Leslie Russell re: EPA view on use of by-product fluosilicic (sic) acid as low cost source of fluoride to water authorities. March 30, 1983.

26 Connett Michael. The Phosphate Fertilizer Industry: An Environmental Overview.Fluoride Action Network. May 2003. Retrieved from http://www.fluoridealert.org/phosphate/overview.htm. Accessed on 7/22/07.

27 Hirzy, W. Press releases. Fluoride 26:279-281, 1993; Fluoride 30:258-259, 1997.

28 http://www.scorecard.org

29 Teotia SPS, Teotia M. Dental Caries: A Disorder of High Fluoride And Low Dietary Calcium Interactions (30 years of Personal Research), Fluoride, 1994 Apr, 27:2, 59-66.

30 Szpunar SM, Eklund SA, Burt BA, Sugar consumption and caries risk in schoolchildren with low caries experience, Community Dent Oral Epidemiol, 1995 Jun, 23(3), 142-146.

31 Riordan PJ. Fluoride supplements for young children: an analysis of the literature focusing on benefits and risks, Community Dentistry & Oral Epidemiology 27(1):72-83, 1999

32 Shulman JD, Wells LM. (1997). Acute fluoride toxicity from ingesting home-use dental products in children, birth to 6 years of age. Journal of Public Health Dentistry 57: 150-8.

33 http://www.fluoridealert.org

34 http://www.fluoridealert.org

35 http://www.fluoridealert.org

36 http://www.fluoridealert.org

37 http://www.fluoridealert.org

38 http://www.fluoridealert.org

Chapter 15
1 World Health Organization. Country profiles of environmental burden of disease: United States of America. Retrieved from http://www.who.int/quantifying_ehimpacts/national/countryprofile/en/index.html. Accessed on 6/14/07.

Chapter Notes

2 Balk, Sophie J et al. Environmental History- Taking.
3 Balk, Sophie J et al. Environmental History- Taking.
4 Lanphear. Lead. New England Journal of Medicine (vol 348, p 1517)
5 Needleman, Herbert. Neurotoxicol. Teratol., 24, 711. 2002.
6 Balk, Sophie J et al. Environmental History- Taking.
7 Balk, Sophie J et al. Environmental History- Taking.
8 Walsh, Bill. Healthy Building Network. Formaldehyde & Kids: Sleep Well.
Retrieved from the healthy building network at
http://www.healthybuilding.net/news/070530sleep_well.html. Accessed
on 8/20/07.
9 http://www.healthybuilding.net/
10 Tambulini, G. et al. Childrens Health and environment: A review of
evidence. European Environment Agency. Environmental issue report. No.
29. Accessed on 1/25/06 at www.euro.who.int/document/e75518.pdf.
11 Balk, Sophie J et al. Environmental History- Taking.
12 NASA. How To Grow Fresh Air.
13 Hirschorn, Joel and Oldenburg, Kirsten V. "Prosperity Without
Pollution". 1991
14 Spring 2002 Edition of CCA Newsletter Partners "Cleaning Without
Toxic Chemicals"
15 http://www.non-toxic.info/Health_Statistics.htm
16 Chec's HealtheHouse,the resource for Environmental Health Risks
Affecting Your Children.
http://www.checnet.org/healthehouse/education/articles-
detail.asp?Main_ID=649
17 Consumer Product Safety Commission. "Chemicals Commonly Found
in the Home"
18 EPA, 1985
19 US Poison Control Centers
20 Chec's HealtheHouse,the resource for Environmental Health Risks
Affecting Your Children.
http://www.checnet.org/healthehouse/education/articles-
detail.asp?Main_ID=649
21 National Resources Council. 1977, 1999
22 Cao, Xinde, Ma, Lena, Tu, Cong. Antioxidative responses to arsenic in
the arsenic-hyperaccumulator Chinese brake fern (Pteris vittata L.).
Environmental Pollution. 128 (2004) 317-325.
23 Healthy Building website.
http://www.healthybuilding.net/arsenic/hbn_wood_factsheet.html
24 Healthy Building website.
25 Cao, Xinde, Ma, Lena, Tu, Cong. Atioxidative responses to arsenic in
the arsenic-hyperaccumulator Chinese brake fern (Pteris vittata L.).
Environmental Pollution. 128 (2004) 317-325.
26 Janssen Sarah. Brominated Flame Retardants: Rising Levels of
Concern. Healthcare without Harm. June 2005. Retrieved from
www.noharm.org. Accessed on 5/14/07.
Houlihan Jane, Brody Charlotte and Schwan Bryony. Not Too Pretty:
Phthalates, Beauty Products, and the FDA. July 8, 2002.

27 Janssen Sarah. Brominated Flame Retardants: Rising Levels of Concern. Healthcare without Harm. June 2005. Retrieved from www.noharm.org. Accessed on 5/14/07.
Houlihan Jane, Brody Charlotte and Schwan Bryony. Not Too Pretty: Phthalates, Beauty Products, and the FDA. July 8, 2002.
28 Groups demand ban on all forms of toxic fire-retardant PBDEs :Legal complaint highlights gaping loopholes in proposed regulations. February 19, 2007 TORONTO, Canada. Retrieved from http://www.davidsuzuki.org/latestnews/dsfnews02190702.asp. Accessed on 5/14/07.
29 Janssen Sarah. Brominated Flame Retardants: Rising Levels of Concern. Healthcare without Harm. June 2005. Retrieved from www.noharm.org. Accessed on 5/14/07.
Houlihan Jane, Brody Charlotte and Schwan Bryony. Not Too Pretty: Phthalates, Beauty Products, and the FDA. July 8, 2002.
30 US Environmental Protection Agency. Office of Pollution Prevention and Toxics. Polybrominated diphenylethers (PBDEs). Retrieved from http://www.epa.gov/oppt/pbde/. Accessed on 5/14/07.
31 US Environmental Protection Agency. Office of Pollution Prevention and Toxics. Polybrominated diphenylethers (PBDEs). Retrieved from http://www.epa.gov/oppt/pbde/. Accessed on 5/14/07.
32 Ken Cook, EWG, May 4, 2007 letter to Dr. David Acheson, Assistant Commissioner for Food Protection. U.S. Food and Drug Administration
33 Groups demand ban on all forms of toxic fire-retardant PBDEs :Legal complaint highlights gaping loopholes in proposed regulations. February 19, 2007 TORONTO, Canada. Retrieved from http://www.davidsuzuki.org/latestnews/dsfnews02190702.asp. Accessed on 5/14/07.
34 Computer Take-Back Campaign. Brominated Flame Retardants in Dust on Computers: The Case for Safer Chemicals and Better Computer Design. Retrieved from http://www.computertakeback.com/the_problem/bfr.cfm. Accessed on 5/14/07.
35 Sugiura-Ogasawara M, Ozaki Y, Sonta S, Makino T, Suzumori K. Exposure to bisphenol A is associated with recurrent miscarriage. Human Reproduction 2005; 20(8):2325-9
36 Janssen Sarah. Brominated Flame Retardants: Rising Levels of Concern. Healthcare without Harm. June 2005. Retrieved from www.noharm.org. Accessed on 5/14/07.
Houlihan Jane, Brody Charlotte and Schwan Bryony. Not Too Pretty: Phthalates, Beauty Products, and the FDA. July 8, 2002.
37 Janssen Sarah. Brominated Flame Retardants: Rising Levels of Concern. Healthcare without Harm. June 2005. Retrieved from www.noharm.org. Accessed on 5/14/07.
Houlihan Jane, Brody Charlotte and Schwan Bryony. Not Too Pretty: Phthalates, Beauty Products, and the FDA. July 8, 2002.
38 Gouveia-Vigeant, Tami and Tickner, Joel. Toxic Chemicals and Childhood Cancer : A Review of the Evidence. Lowell Center for Sustainable Production. University of Massachusetts Lowell. May, 2003.

39 Baue, Williams. Pesticides in Your Home. Childrens Health Environmental Coalition. 8/21/03. Retrieved from http://www.checnet.org/healthehouse/education/articles-detail.asp?Main_ID=439.

40 Mills PK, Yang R. Regression analysis of pesticide use and breast cancer incidence in California. Latinas. J Environ Health. 68(6):15-22 . 2006.

41 (U.S. Environmental Protection Agency 2000, 2002), (Casida and Quistad 2004).

42 (Landrigan 2001; Landrigan et al. 1999; May 2000; Physicians for Social Responsibility 1995; Pope 1999; Slotkin 1999, 2004; Weiss et al. 2004).

43 Slotkin, Theodore, Charlotte A Tate, Ian T Ryde, Edward D Levin, Frederic J Seidler. Organophosphate Insecticides Target the Serotonergic System in Developing Rat Brain Regions: Disparate Effects of Diazinon and Parathion at Doses Spanning the Threshold for Cholinesterase Inhibition. Environmental Health Perspectives. Volume 114, Number 10, October 2006.

44 Kilburn, K.H. and Thornton, J.C.: Protracted neurotoxicity from chlordane sprayed to kill termites. Environ. Health Perspect. 103(7-8): 690-694, 1995.

Chapter 16

1 http://www.thegreenguide.com

2 http://www.thegreenguide.com

3 Ecology Center Website. Adverse Health Effects of Plastics. Retrieved from http://www.ecologycenter.org/factsheets/plastichealtheffects.html. Accessed on6/7/07.

4 World Health Organization. Global Assessment of the State-of-the-Science of Endocrine Disruptors. 2002.

5 Frustaci A, Magnavita N, Chimenti C, Caldarulo M, Sabbioni E, Pietra R, Cellini C, Possati GF, Maseri A. Department of Cardiology, Catholic University, Rome, Italy. "Marked elevation of myocardial trace elements in idiopathic dilated cardiomyopathy compared with secondary cardiac dysfunction." From: J Am Coll Cardiol 1999 May;33(6):1578-83

6 Rick Hind and Charlie Kay of Greenpeace from the documentary "Blue Vinyl"

7 George Lucier, PhD, Former Director of the Environmental Toxicology Program of the National Institute of Heatlh. From the Documentary "Blue Vinyl"

8 Interview of Dr. P. Brandt-Lauf from Columbia University's Department of Environmental Medicine. From the Documentary "Blue Vinyl"

9 The International Association of Firefighters

10 Kremer, Andrea. Cradle to Grave: The Life Cycle of Styrofoam. Race, Poverty, and the Urban Environment. Professor Raquel Pinderhughes. Urban Studies Program. San Francisco State University. Spring 2003.

11 Kremer, Andrea. Cradle to Grave: The Life Cycle of Styrofoam. Race, Poverty, and the Urban Environment. Professor Raquel Pinderhughes. Urban Studies Program. San Francisco State University. Spring 2003.

12 Kremer, Andrea. Cradle to Grave: The Life Cycle of Styrofoam. Race, Poverty, and the Urban Environment. Professor Raquel Pinderhughes. Urban Studies Program. San Francisco State University. Spring 2003.
13
http://www.ourstolenfuture.org/newscience/oncompounds/bisphenola/b pauses.htm
14 vom Saal, F and Hughes, C. An Extensive New Literature Concerning Low-Dose Effects of Bisphenol A Shows the Need for a New Risk Assessment. Environmental Health Perspectives. Volume 113, Number 8, August 2005.
15 vom Saal and Hughes, 2005.
16 Maffini MV, Rubin BS, Sonnenschein C, Soto AM. Endocrine disruptors and reproductive health: The case of bisphenol A. Molecular and Cellular Endocrinology 2006, 25:179-186
17 Gibson, Rachel.. Toxic Baby Bottles. 2/27/2007. Environment California Research and Policy Center: Scientific Study Finds Leaching Chemicals in Clear Plastic Baby Bottles. Retrieved from http://www.environmentcalifornia.org/reports/environmental-health/environmental-health-reports/toxic-baby-bottles#LbBM-jO8vN4knBwWoS8zww. Accessed on 5/16/07.
18 vom Saal and Hughes, 2005.
19 http://www.thegreenguide.com
20 Health Care Without Harm. "Pretty Nasty: Phthalates in European Cosmetic Products". Sweden. 2002
21 Health Care Without Harm. Aggregate Exposures to Phthalates in Humans. July 2002.
22 Environment California Research and Policy Center. StopToxic Toys: Toxics Fact Sheet. Retrieved from http://www.environmentcalifornia.org/environmental-health/stop-toxic-toys/toxics-fact-sheet. Accessed on 5/16/07.
23 Environment California Research and Policy Center. StopToxic Toys: Toxics Fact Sheet. Retrieved from http://www.environmentcalifornia.org/environmental-health/stop-toxic-toys/toxics-fact-sheet. Accessed on 5/16/07.
24 Toloken, Steve. "Federal Panel Takes Another Look at DEHP" Plastics News. 10/13/05
25 Health Care Without Harm. Aggregate Exposures to Phthalates in Humans. July 2002.
26 Davis, Devra. When Smoke Ran Like Water, p180.
27 Blount, et al. "Levels of Seven Urinary Phthalate Metabolites in a Human Reference Population," Environmental Health Perspectives, Vol. 108 No. 10. October 2000.
28 Environment California Research and Policy Center. StopToxic Toys: Toxics Fact Sheet. Retrieved from http://www.environmentcalifornia.org/environmental-health/stop-toxic-toys/toxics-fact-sheet. Accessed on 5/16/07.
29 Gibson, Rachel. Committee Passes Legislation to Ban Phthalates from Baby Products: Press Release from Environment California. 5/9/07. Retrieved from

http://www.environmentcalifornia.org/newsroom/environmental-
health/environmental-health-news/assembly-health-committee-passes-
legislation-to-ban-phthalates-from-baby-products. Accessed on 5/17/07.
30 Institute for Agriculture and Trade Policy. Smart Plastics Guide:
Healthier Food Uses of Plastics for Parents and Children.Minneapolis, MN.
October 2006. Retrieved from www.IATP.org/foodandhealth. Accessed on
6/7/07.
31 Institute for Agriculture and Trade Policy. Smart Plastics Guide:
Healthier Food Uses of Plastics for Parents and Children.Minneapolis, MN.
October 2006. Retrieved from www.IATP.org/foodandhealth. Accessed on
6/7/07.

Chapter 17
1 Campaign for Safe Cosmetics Website: http://www.safecosmetics.org
2 www.cosmeticsdatabase.com
3 Campaign for Safe Cosmetics. Frequently Asked Questions About 1,4-
Dioxane. Retrieved from http://www.safecosmetics.org/faqs/dioxane.cfm.
Accessed on 5/17/07.
4 Campaign for Safe Cosmetics Website:
5 Environmental Working Group - June 2004.
6 CIR 2004. Environmental Working Group - June 2000.
7 Houlihan, Jane, Charlotte Brody, and Bryony Schwan. Not Too Pretty:
Phthalates, Beauty Products, and the FDA. Environmental Working Group.
July 8, 2002.
8 Healthcare Without Harm. Pretty Nasty: Phthalates in European
Cosmetic Products. November 2002.
9 Darbre P D, Aljarrah A, Miller W R, Coldham N G, Sauer M J, and Pope
G S. Concentrations of Parabens in Human Breast Tumours. Journal of
Applied Toxicology. Vol 24, 2004, p. 5-13.
10 Pediatric Forum. Archives Ped Adol Medicne 2002
11 Tiwary CM. Premature Sexual Development in Children Following the
Use of Estrogen of Placenta Containing Hair Products. Clin Pediatrics.
1998;37:733-739.
12 Somogyi, L. et. al. 1994
13 Wolff, Peggy. Synthetic Fragrance and Health. 5/8/07. Retrieved from
http://www.noharm.org/us/nurses#grants. Accessed on 5/16/07.
14 Anderson, R. & J. Anderson. "Acute Toxic Effects of Fragrance
Products", Archives of Environmental Health March-April, 1998. 53 (2),
138-146.

Chapter 18
1 Wikipedia
2 National Academy of Sciences. Health Risks from Exposure to Low Levels
of Ionizing Radiation: BEIR VII Phase 2. National Academies Press. 2006.
3 Tice R and Hook G, Integrated Laboratory Systems in North Carolina,
1998.
Dr. Joseph Roti Roti of Washington University in St. Louis in 2000.
4 Hardell O, Carlberg M, Söderqvist F, Mild KH and Morgan LL. Long-term
use of cellular phones and brain tumours - increased risk associated with

use for > 10 years. Occup Environ Med. Published Online First: 4 April 2007. Retrieved from http://oem.bmj.com/cgi/content/abstract/oem.2006.029751v1. Accessed on 8/21/07.

5 Ahlbom A, Day N, Feychting M, Roman E, Skinner, J, Dockerty J, et al. 2000. A pooled analysis of magnetic fields and childhood leukaemia. Br J Cancer 83: 692–698.

6 Hardell O, Carlberg M, Söderqvist F, Mild KH and Morgan LL. Long-term use of cellular phones and brain tumours - increased risk associated with use for > 10 years. Occup Environ Med. Published Online First: 4 April 2007. Retrieved from http://oem.bmj.com/cgi/content/abstract/oem.2006.029751v1. Accessed on 8/21/07.

7 Chia SE, Chia HP, Tan JS. Prevalence of headache among handheld cellular telephone users in Singapore: a community study. Environmental Health Perspectives Volume 108, Number 11, November 2000 (p. 1059-62)

8 Aalto S, Haarala C, Brück A, Sipilä H, Hämäläinen H, Rinne JO. Mobile phone affects cerebral blood flow in humans. J Cereb Blood Flow Metab. 2006 Jul;26(7):885-90. Epub 2006 Feb 22.

9 Salford LG, Brun AE, Eberhardt JL, Malmgren L, and Persson BRR. Mobile Phone Exposure Causes Brain Damage in Rats Environmental Health Perspectives 111:881-883].

10 Ozguner F, Altinbas A, Ozaydin M, Dogan A, Vural H, Kisioglu AN, Cesur G, Yildirim NG. Mobile phone-induced myocardial oxidative stress: protection by a novel antioxidant agent caffeic acid phenethyl ester. Toxicol Ind Health. 2005 Oct;21(9):223-30.,

Ozguner F, Oktem F, Armagan A, Yilmaz R, Koyu A, Demirel R, Vural H, Uz E.Comparative analysis of the protective effects of melatonin and caffeic acid phenethyl ester (CAPE) on mobile phone-induced renal impairment in rat. Mol Cell Biochem. 2005 Aug;276(1-2):31-7.

11 Maisch, Don. Medical Warnings Needed on DECT cordless phone use. J. Aust. Coll. Nutr. & Env. Med. 25(2). August 2006.

12 Campion, EW, associate editor of NEJM. Editorial. New England Journal of Medicine (337:1) July 3, 1997

13 NIEHS EMF-RAPID Program Staff. National Institute of Environmental Health Sciences. National Institutes of Health. "Health Effects from Exposure to Power-Line Frequency Electric and Magnetic Fields." May 4, 1999. World Health Organization. Electromagnetic fields and public health: extremely low frequency fields and cancer.

14 California Department of Health Servicea. An Evaluation of the Possible Risks From Electric and Magnetic Fields (EMFs) From Power Lines, Internal Wiring, Electrical Occupations and Appliances.

15 H.K. Florig[1], M. Henrion[2], A.R. Sheppard[3], B. Bernstein[4] and K. Soohoo Annual Review of Research on the Biological Effects of Electric and Magnetic Fields from the Generation, Delivery and Use of Electricity, San Antonio, Texas, USA, November 19-21, 1996. World Health Organization. http://www.who.int/mediacentre/factsheets/fs322/en/index.html)

Chapter Notes

16 California Electric and Magnetic Fields Program. Frequently Asked Questions About Magnetic Fields and Homes.
17 Dr. Ken Rothman of Eidemiology Resources, Inc. in Newton, Mass, 1998.

Chapter 19

1 Adapted with permission from Luna-Pinsker, Claire. "Please send my son home exhausted!" retrieved from
www.musicoflovewriter.com<http://www.musicoflovewriter.com/
2 Kanner, Leo. Autistic Disturbances of Affective Contact. Nervous Child. 1943. VOl 2. p217-250.
3 Fox, Maggie. Autism Prevalence in U.S. Greater Than Previous Estimates. Reuters Health Information. 2007. Retrieved from www.medscape.com/viewarticle/551907. Accessed on 2/14/07.
4 DDS, Autistic Spectrum Disorders, Changes in the California Caseload: 1999-2002
5 Agency for Toxic Substances and Disease Registry. ToxFAQs for Mercury, April 1999 Retrieved from http://www.atsdr.cdc.gov/tfacts46.html. Accessed on April 9, 2007
6 Olmstead, Dan. "The Age of Autism: A Pretty Big Secret" December 7, 2005. United Press International Lancaster, PA
7 Olmstead, Dan. "The Age of Autism: The Amish anomaly" April 18, 2005. United Press International Lancaster, PA
8 Kirby, David. Thoughtful House presentation. Retrieved from www.thoughtfulhouse.org. Accessed on 4/10/07.
9 Jepson, Bryan. Thoughtful House Presentation. Retrieved from www.thoughtfulhouse.org. Accessed on 4/10/07.
10 Mumper, Elizabeth M.D. Thoughtful House Presentation. Retrieved from http://www.thoughtfulhouse.org/0405-conf-emumper.htm. Accessed on 4/12/07.
11 James, S.J. et al.: Metabolic biomarkers of increased oxidative stress and impaired methylation capacity in children with autism. Am. J. Clin. Nutr. 80, 1611-1617 2004.
12 Hornig M, Chian D, Lipkin WI "Neurotoxic effects of postnatal thimerosal are mouse strain-dependent (advance online publication)" Molec Psychiatry.8 June 2004.
13 Pichichero et al: Mercury concentrations and metabolism in infants receiving vaccines containing thiomersal: a descriptive study. Lancet 360, 1737-1741 2002
14 Haley, Boyd E. Toxic Overload: Assessing the Role of Mercury in Autism. Mothering. Volume 115, November/December 2002 Retrieved from
http://www.mothering.com/articles/growing_child/vaccines/toxic.html. Accessed on 4/12/07.
15 James, S.J. et al.: Metabolic biomarkers of increased oxidative stress and impaired methylation capacity in children with autism. Am. J. Clin. Nutr. 80, 1611-1617 2004.
16 Kirby, David. Evidence of Harm. St. Martin's Press. 2005.
17 1982 Federal Register.

18 Kirby, David. Evidence of Harm. St. Martin's Press. 2005.
19 Kirby, David. Evidence of Harm. St. Martin's Press. 2005.
20 Jepson, Bryan. Thoughtful House Presentation. Retrieved from www.thoughtfulhouse.org. Accessed on 4/10/07.
21 Kirby, David. Evidence of Harm. St. Martin's Press. 2005.
22 Kirby, David. Evidence of Harm. St. Martin's Press. 2005.
23 Burbacher T, et al. Comparison of blood and brain mercury levels in infant
monkeys exposed to methylmercury or vaccines containing thimerosal. Environmental Health Perspectives, 2005 Aug:113(8):1015-21.
24 Subcommittee on Human Rights and Wellness, Mercury in Medicine Report, United States Congress
25 Kirby, David. Thoughtful House presentation. Retrieved from www.thoughtfulhouse.org. Accessed on 4/10/07.
26 VAERS Data. www.cancerdecisions.com , 6/17/07
27 http://www.gotmercury.org/
28 Turtle Island Restoration Network
29 http://www.epa.gov/air/mercuryrule/charts.htm
30 Lang, Martha. (Telephone Interview)
31 Environmental Working Group. BodyBurden: The Pollution in Newborns. *July 14, 2005.*
32 Datz, Todd. A Silent Pandemic: Industrial Chemicals Are Impairing the Brain Development of Children Worldwide. Nov 7, 2006. Harvard School of Public Health. Boston, MA. Retrieved from Harvard.edu. Accessed on 3/30/07.
33 Heavy metals may be implicated in autism. New Scientist. issue 2553. 30 May 2006, page 21.
34 Bradstreet, J et al.: A case control study of mercury burden in children with autistic spectrum disorders. J. Am. Phys. Surg. 8,76-79 2003
35 Buttar, Rashid A. Autism, The Misdiagnosis of Our Future Generations. Testimony: Autsism Spectrum Disorders: An Update of Federal Government Initiatives and Revolutionary New Treatments of Neurodevelopmental Diseases. May 7, 2004. Retrieved from www.generaionrescue.org. Accessed on 4/10/07.
36 James, S.J. et al.: Metabolic biomarkers of increased oxidative stress and impaired methylation capacity in children with autism. Am. J. Clin. Nutr. 80, 1611-1617 2004.
37 The Childhood Autism Risks from Genetics and the Environment study: Tracing the Origins of Autism, 2006
38 Ashwood, Paul PhD. Thoughtful House Presentation.

Chapter 20
1 Svare, et al. Mercury Vapor Testing. Journal of Dental Research. 1981. 60 (9): 1668-71
2 Nylander et al. Swedish Dental Journal. Vol 11. 1987. 179-187
3 Vimy MJ, Hooper DF, King WW, Lorscheider FL. Mercury from Maternal "Silver"Tooth Fillings in Sheep and Human Breast Milk: A Source of Neonatal Exposure. Biological Trace Element Research. 56. 143-52. 1997

4 Lorscheider et al. Mercury Exposure From Silver Tooth Fillings: Emerging Evidence Questions a Traditional Dental Paradigm. FASEB Journal. April 1995
5 Centers for Disease Control and Prevention. 2001.
6 Huggins, Hal. Telephone interview conducted on 9/7.07.
7 Huggins, Hal. Telephone interview conducted on 9/7.07.
8 Huggins, Hal. Telephone interview conducted on 9/7.07.

Chapter 21
1 A Rainbow A Day and Food Studies Institute, 2004. Information presented by Ioana Razi, MD on Thursday, June 28 at "Food as Medicine" Conference in Baltimore, MD
2 Kritchevsky D. Diet, nutrition, and cancer: the role of fiber. Cancer. 1986;58:1830-6
3 Dr. Joseph Pizzorno, President Emeritus of Bastyr University and Editor of Integrative Medicine: A Clinician's Journal. Information presented at "Food as Medicine" Conference in Baltimore, MD June 2007.

Chapter 22
1 Landrigan Philip J., Paul J. Lioy, George Thurston, Gertrud Berkowitz, L.C. Chen, Steven N. Chillrud, Stephen H. Gavett, Panos G. Georgopoulos, Alison S. Geyh, Stephen Levin, Frederica Perera, Stephen M. Rappaport, Christopher Small, and the NIEHS World Trade Center Working Group. Workgroup Report: Health and Environmental Consequences of the World Trade Center Disaster.
Environmental Health Perspectives Volume 112, Number 6, May 2004. Retrieved from
http://www.ehponline.org/members/2004/6702/6702.html. Accessed on 6/3/07.
2 Herbert Robin, Luft Benjamin, Markowitz Steven, Udasin Iris, Harrison Denise, Stein Diane, Todd Andrew, Enright Paul, Stellman Jeanne Mager, Landrigan Philip J, and Levin Stephen M. The World Trade Center Disaster and the Health of Workers: Five-Year Assessment of a Unique Medical Screening Program. Environmental Health Perspectives Volume 114, Number 12, December 2006.
3 Root David E. Downtown Medical: A Detoxification Program for WTC Responders. Fire Engineering: Training the Fire Service for 126 years. June 2003. Retrieved from www.FireEngineering.com. Accessed on 6/3/07.
4 Rachinow, Jonnie. Treatment of World Trade Center Exposures: Results from Detoxification. Presentation Abstract. Third International Conference on Chemical Contamination and Human Detoxification. Hunter College. New York, NY. Septemeber 22-23, 2005.
5 Foundation for Advancements in Science and Education website. Detoxification.
http://fasenet.org/environment.html
6 Foundation for Advancements in Science and Education website. Detoxification.
http://fasenet.org/environment.html

7 Root David E. Downtown Medical: A Detoxification Program for WTC Responders. Fire Engineering: Training the Fire Service for 126 years. June 2003. Retrieved from www.FireEngineering.com. Accessed on 6/3/07.
8 Root David E. Downtown Medical: A Detoxification Program for WTC Responders. Fire Engineering: Training the Fire Service for 126 years. June 2003. Retrieved from www.FireEngineering.com. Accessed on 6/3/07.

Chapter 23
1 Brody J. Breast Cancer and the Environment: Science News From Silent Spring Institute. July 2004
2 American Cancer Society
3 Bau, William.. Social Investment Forum Trends Report Tracks Rises and Falls of Socially Responsible Investing. January 26, 2006. Retrieved from http://www.socialfunds.com/news/article.cgi/1913.html. Accessed on 7/11/07.
4 Newman, Nell. Newman's Own Organics: A Guide to the Good Life. p89.
5 Kushner Harold S. Living a Life That Matters.: Resolving the Conflict Between Conscience and Success. Borzoi Book published by Alfred Knopf. New York. 2001.
6 Landrigan Philip, Garg Anjali, and Droller Daniel B.J. Assessing the effects of endocrine disruptors in the National Children's Study. Environmental Health Perspectives. 111:1678-82. 2003.

I*ndex*

Index

Index

237

Professional Speaking Services

Teresa Holler, author of *Cardiology Essentials* and *Holler for Your Health: Be the Key to a Healthy Family*, is a highly regarded speaker who believes it is time we stop treating and start preventing disease. Her keynotes are ideal for women's groups, health expos, college campuses, corporate wellness programs, and partner programs. Send an email to **speak@holler4health.com** for more information.

A Few Words From the
President of the National Speakers Association

"Teresa captivated the audience with her ideas on how to prevent disease. Her suggestions were simple, practical, and can be implemented immediately. Her health-saving strategies are sure to impact the lives of all who are fortunate enough to hear her message. Every person, and especially every parent, needs to hear her speak. It will be life-changing for those who do."

-Mark LeBlanc, Author of *Growing Your Business* and President of the National Speakers Association

Continuing Medical Education

Medical Professionals interested in learning more about environmental health, functional medicine and truly effective disease prevention while earning CME credits should visit **www.harborhealthseminars.com**

Give the Gift of Health to Your Loved Ones and Friends

Friends Don't Let Friends Raise a Child without Reading This Book: Makes a Great Baby Shower Gift!

Order additional copies from your local bookstore, amazon.com, or directly from the author at **www.holler4health.com**

Printed in the United States
202310BV00004B/1-120/P